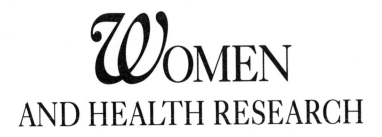

# WOMEN
## AND HEALTH RESEARCH

ETHICAL AND LEGAL ISSUES OF
INCLUDING WOMEN IN CLINICAL STUDIES

VOLUME I

Anna C. Mastroianni, Ruth Faden, and Daniel Federman, *Editors*

Committee on the Ethical and Legal Issues
Relating to the Inclusion of Women in Clinical Studies

Division of Health Sciences Policy

INSTITUTE OF MEDICINE

NATIONAL ACADEMY PRESS
Washington, D.C. 1994

**National Academy Press • 2101 Constitution Avenue, N.W. • Washington, D.C. 20418**

NOTICE: The project that is the subject of this report was approved by the Governing Board of the National Research Council, whose members are drawn from the councils of the National Academy of Sciences, the National Academy of Engineering, and the Institute of Medicine. The members of the committee responsible for the report were chosen for their special competencies and with regard for appropriate balance.

This report has been reviewed by a group other than the authors according to procedures approved by a Report Review Committee consisting of members of the National Academy of Sciences, the National Academy of Engineering, and the Institute of Medicine.

The Institute of Medicine was chartered in 1970 by the National Academy of Sciences to enlist distinguished members of the appropriate professions in the examination of policy matters pertaining to the health of the public. In this, the Institute acts under both the Academy's 1863 congressional charter responsibility to be an adviser to the federal government and its own initiative in identifying issues of medical care, research, and education. Dr. Kenneth I. Shine is president of the Institute of Medicine.

This project was funded by the Office of Research on Women's Health of the National Institutes of Health (Contract No. NO1-OD-2-2119) with supplemental support provided by The Ford Foundation (Grant No. 935-1335). Syntex (U.S.A.), Inc. and the Institute of Medicine also provided support for this project.

**Library of Congress Cataloging-in-Publication Data**

Women and health research : ethical and legal issues of including
    women in clinical studies / Anna C. Mastroianni, Ruth Faden, and
    Daniel Federman, editors ; Committee on the Ethical and Legal Issues
    Relating to the Inclusion of Women in Clinical Studies, Division of
    Health Sciences Policy, Institute of Medicine.
        p.  cm.
    Includes bibliographical references and index.
    ISBN 0-309-04992-X
      1. Women—Health and hygiene—Research—Moral and ethical aspects.
    2. Human experimentation in medicine—Moral and ethical aspects.
    3. Human experimentation in medicine—Law and legislation.
    4. United States. National Institutes of Health Revitalization Act
    of 1993. I. Mastroianni, Anna C. II. Faden, Ruth R.
    III. Federman, Daniel D., 1928-   . IV. Institute of Medicine
    (U.S.). Committee on the Ethical and Legal Issues Relating to the
    Inclusion of Women in Clinical Studies.
      [DNLM: 1. Ethics, Medical. 2. Clinical Protocols. 3. Women's
    Health. 4. Research—United States—legislation. W 20.5 W872
    1994]
    R853.H8W66   1994
    174'.28—dc20
    DNLM/DLC
    for Library of Congress                     93-50549
                                          CIP

Printed in the United States of America.

The serpent has been a symbol of long life, healing, and knowledge among almost all cultures and religions since the beginning of recorded history. The image adopted as a logotype by the Institute of Medicine is based on a relief carving from ancient Greece, now held by the Staalichemuseen in Berlin.

# COMMITTEE ON THE ETHICAL AND LEGAL ISSUES RELATING TO THE INCLUSION OF WOMEN IN CLINICAL STUDIES

**RUTH FADEN**, Ph.D., M.P.H. (*Co-chair*), Professor and Director, Program in Law, Ethics, and Health, School of Hygiene and Public Health, The Johns Hopkins University, and Senior Research Scholar, Kennedy Institute of Ethics, Georgetown University

**DANIEL FEDERMAN**, M.D.* (*Co-chair*), Professor of Medicine, Dean of Medical Education, Harvard Medical School

**ANITA ALLEN**, J.D., Ph.D., Professor of Law, Georgetown University Law Center

**HORTENSIA AMARO**, Ph.D., Professor of Social and Behavioral Sciences, School of Public Health, Boston University School of Medicine

**KAREN H. ANTMAN**, M.D., Chief, Division of Medical Oncology, Columbia-Presbyterian Medical Center, New York

**LIONEL D. EDWARDS**, M.D., Assistant Vice President and Senior Director of Therapeutic Research Operations II, Hoffmann-La Roche, Inc., Nutley, New Jersey

**ANN BARRY FLOOD**, Ph.D., Director of Policy Studies and Associate Professor at the Center for the Evaluative Clinical Sciences, Dartmouth Medical School

**SHIRIKI K. KUMANYIKA**, Ph.D., M.P.H., Professor of Epidemiology, Center for Biostatistics and Epidemiology, Pennsylvania State College of Medicine

**RUTH MACKLIN**, Ph.D.*, Professor of Epidemiology and Social Medicine, Albert Einstein College of Medicine

**DONALD R. MATTISON**, M.D., Dean, Graduate School of Public Health, University of Pittsburgh

**CHARLES R. McCARTHY**, Ph.D., Senior Research Fellow, Kennedy Institute of Ethics, Georgetown University, and Retired Director of the Office of Protection from Research Risks, National Institutes of Health, Richmond, Virginia

**CURTIS MEINERT**, Ph.D., Director, Center for Clinical Trials, Professor of Epidemiology and Biostatistics, School of Hygiene and Public Health, The Johns Hopkins University

**KAREN H. ROTHENBERG**, J.D., M.P.A., Professor of Law, Director, Law and Healthcare Programs, University of Maryland School of Law

*Member, Institute of Medicine

**ANTHONY R. SCIALLI**, M.D., Director, Residency Program, Georgetown University Medical Center, and Director, Reproductive Toxicology Center, Columbia Hospital for Women Medical Center, Washington, D.C.

**SHELDON J. SEGAL**, Ph.D.*, Distinguished Scientist, The Population Council, New York

**WALTER J. WADLINGTON**, LL.B.*, Professor of Law and of Legal Medicine, University of Virginia Law School

Study Staff

**ANNA C. MASTROIANNI**, Study Director
**RUTH ELLEN BULGER**, Division Director (until August 1993)
**VALERIE P. SETLOW**, Division Director (from August 1993)
**ELIZABETH MEYER BOBBY**, Research Associate
**THELMA L. COX**, Project Assistant
**PHILOMINA MAMMEN**, Administrative Assistant

---

*Member, Institute of Medicine

# Preface

A perception has grown in recent years that biomedical research has focused more on the health problems of men than on those of women, and that women have been denied access to advances in medical diagnosis and therapy as a result of being excluded from clinical studies. The atmosphere surrounding this perception is one of conflict and change. There has been conflict between those who hold the perception and those who do not, and between concerns about protecting women from the risks of research participation and about their access to its potential benefits. At the same time, there have been substantial changes in public opinion about the desirability of participating in research, and equally marked changes in federal research policies. The need to illuminate the conflicts and evaluate the changes led to the present study.

The National Institutes of Health (NIH) Revitalization Act of June 1993 introduced new requirements for the inclusion of women and minorities in federally funded clinical studies except where specific criteria for the exclusion of these groups can be satisfied. Congress intended the Act to be responsive to the serious allegations of "underrepresentation" of women in clinical research, and to be corrective of any disparities. Most scientists

---

The final manuscript of this report was delivered to the sponsoring federal agency, the Office of Research on Women's Health of the National Institutes of Health, on November 30, 1993, in accordance with contractual obligations.

support these objectives, yet many have expressed grave concerns that the strategies outlined in the Act for attaining these objectives may be seriously flawed. The detection of significant differences in response among subgroups, many have argued, generally requires clinical studies that are large, time-consuming, and expensive—in many cases, prohibitively so. Because cost was specified as an unacceptable criterion for exclusion, the need to design studies that comply with the new legislation may ultimately result in fewer clinical studies being done on anyone.

It is not surprising that the requirements specified in the NIH Revitalization Act are contentious. The inclusion of women in clinical studies raises a mélange of often conflicting ethical, legal, scientific, and social traditions and concerns. Several efforts have been made to sort out these difficult issues and to shape an appropriate policy of inclusion. In March 1991, at NIH's request, the Institute of Medicine (IOM) convened a meeting at which a panel was asked to (a) assess the adequacy of the existing knowledge base for formulating gender-specific hypotheses and (b) consider the advisability of conducting a study to explore further women's participation in clinical studies. The panel concluded that important unresolved problems and questions remained. Given changes in societal attitudes and advances in medical technology, the panel felt a reexamination of existing policies and practices would be productive.

In September 1992, in response to a request from the NIH Office of Research on Women's Health, the IOM convened the Committee on the Ethical and Legal Issues Relating to the Inclusion of Women in Clinical Studies. The 16 members of the committee have backgrounds in bioethics, law, epidemiology and biostatistics, public health policy, obstetrics and gynecology, clinical research, pharmaceutical development, social and behavioral sciences, and clinical evaluative sciences.

The committee's charge was to (a) consider the ethical and legal implications of including women, particularly pregnant women and women of childbearing potential, in clinical studies; (b) provide practical advice for consideration by NIH, institutional review boards, and clinical investigators; and (c) examine known instances of litigation regarding injuries to research subjects and to describe existing legal liabilities and protections. Although the committee was not asked to examine scientific issues related to women's inclusion in clinical studies, the members felt strongly that a basic understanding of both gender-specific physiological differences and methods for clinical study design was essential to its deliberations and to the development of reasoned arguments to support policy recommendations in this area. We have included a summary of the history of women's participation in clinical research to enhance readers' understanding of the origins of controversy and concern on this issue.

As is discussed in the first chapter of this report, the effort to assess the current status of women's participation in clinical studies was frustrated by the lack of systematic information on the gender composition of subject populations. Despite a concerted effort to locate data, firm conclusions regarding the relative participation of women and men in the whole of clinical research could not be drawn.

The members agreed that policy recommendations for the inclusion of women in clinical studies need not depend on proof that women have been "underrepresented" in clinical studies in the past. The fact that existing research guidelines from the Department of Health and Human Services and the Food and Drug Administration presumed that pregnant women and women of childbearing potential should be excluded from clinical studies except in limited circumstances was adequate evidence of a need for new policies. Moreover, an articulation of ethical and legal considerations does not require proof of ethically or legally questionable practices. Our task was to examine ethical standards in the context of American law; the empirical challenge of determining the extent to which these standards are being met still remains.

Recognizing that calls to rectify women's alleged "underrepresentation" in clinical studies were based on concerns about unequal distribution of the benefits of biomedical research, the committee chose to form its analysis around principles of justice. Simply stated, the committee believes that women and men should have the opportunity to participate equally in the benefits and burdens of research. Throughout the course of our deliberations, several distinct appeals to justice in the context of clinical studies took shape. These appeals, described in Chapter 3, guided the composition of each of our arguments and recommendations.

The achievement of the principles of justice outlined in this report will not be without scientific, social, ethical, and legal quandaries and challenges. The committee has attempted to anticipate these difficulties and to illuminate the concerns of all who have an interest in clinical research, including potential subjects, policymakers, members of research review committees, investigators, and the general public. Recent changes in federal research policy are intended to increase women's participation in clinical studies, but we believe further action is needed to achieve true justice throughout clinical research. For pregnant women in particular, the need is great to resolve the controversy concerning their inclusion in clinical studies. It is the committee's sincere hope that those who read this report will gain new insights from our analysis that may be helpful in moving closer toward resolution of the issues surrounding the inclusion of all women in clinical studies.

The committee has tried to weave ethical, legal, social, and scientific threads into a fabric of guidelines for the full inclusion of women in clinical research. We believe that an inclusive approach will help both the subjects of research and the numerous others who indirectly benefit from their participation. We have listened broadly, argued heatedly, and concluded provisionally. Although we represent many different backgrounds, we are nevertheless unanimous in pointing out the critical importance of achieving justice in clinical research and in believing that goal will be furthered by the increased participation of women as subjects, scientists, and policymakers.

Ruth Faden, *Co-chair*
Daniel Federman, *Co-chair*

# Acknowledgments

The committee wishes to express its gratitude to those who prepared background papers: Chloe Bird of the New England Medical Center and Harvard University, Bonnie Ellen Blustein of the University of Wisconsin, Sandra Cassard of the Johns Hopkins University, Elizabeth Fee of the Johns Hopkins University, Vanessa Northington Gamble of the University of Wisconsin, Tracy Johnson of the Society for the Advancement of Women's Health Research, Barbara Lex of Harvard University, Janice Racine Norris of Harvard University, Carol Weisman of the Johns Hopkins University, Elena Yu of San Diego State University, and Ruth Zambrana of the University of California at Los Angeles and the Agency for Health Care Policy and Research.

The committee also thanks those who gave presentations at its workshop: Leslie Benet of the University of California at San Francisco, R. Alta Charo of the University of Wisconsin, Ellen Wright Clayton of Vanderbilt University, Debra DeBruin of the University of Illinois at Chicago, Ellen Flannery and Sanford N. Greenberg of the Washington, D.C., law firm of Covington and Burling, Robert Levine of Yale University, Wendy Mariner of Boston University, Vanessa Merton of Pace University, Janet Mitchell of Harlem Hospital Center and Columbia University, Jonathan Moreno of the State University of New York Health Sciences Center (Brooklyn), John Robertson of the University of Texas, Susan Sherwin of Dalhousie University, Bonnie Steinbock of the State University of New York at Albany, and Diane Stoy of the George Washington University.

Staff at the following organizations were also very helpful: ACT-UP, Center for Women's Policy Studies, Congressional Caucus for Women's Issues, Food and Drug Administration, Food and Drug Law Institute, Institute for Research on Women's Health, National Women's Health Network, Pharmaceutical Manufacturers Association, Society for the Advancement of Women's Health Research, the University of Washington, and the U.S. General Accounting Office. We also thank the products liability attorneys and directors of regulatory affairs at pharmaceutical companies who provided information as their corporate policies allowed. We also appreciate the efforts of the staff at the National Institutes of Health in providing the committee with data.

We owe particular appreciation to Elizabeth Meyer, research associate, who helped organize the committee, provided necessary support throughout the study, and assisted with the research and drafting of the report. We also thank Thelma Cox, project assistant, who helped with meeting planning and logistics, distributed briefing materials, and provided general committee support. Special thanks are owed to Ruth Ellen Bulger, who continued to provide valuable advice after leaving her position as director of the Division of Health Sciences Policy.

We are especially grateful to Beth Kosiak for her organizational insight and editing, and to Deven McGraw for her legal research and drafting contributions to Chapter 6. We also thank Philomina Mammen for assisting in proposal preparation, Kimberly Kasberg Maraviglia for preparing legislative and regulatory analyses, and Gail Spears for collecting agency policies and providing research assistance. Additional thanks are owed to Paul Phelps for editing and improving many sections of the report, to Mike Edington for editing and publication coordination, to Claudia Carl for coordination of the review process, and to Nancy Diener for budgeting guidance.

It would be difficult to express adequately our debt to Anna Mastroianni. As a professional colleague, she made numerous substantive contributions. As study director, she organized the efforts of all those named in these acknowledgments. And throughout, but particularly as we worked to refine our views and reach conclusions, she manifested excellent judgment and inexhaustible patience.

This report truly is a committee document. Members of the committee were dedicated and involved throughout the study, from early drafting through final revisions. All of our colleagues made generous contributions of time, energy, and expert knowledge; their insights and ideas were pivotal in the development of this report.

Ruth Faden, *Co-chair*
Daniel Federman, *Co-chair*

# Contents

# *W*OMEN
## AND HEALTH RESEARCH

# Executive Summary

There is a general perception that biomedical research has not given the same attention to the health problems of women that it has given to those of men, and that women may not have benefited from advances in medical diagnosis and therapy because of their lower rates of participation in clinical studies. These perceived inequities have recently become the focus of public attention and legislative action, as women's health advocates and others challenge the content of the national research agenda. Recent policy responses to these perceptions present very real challenges to Institutional Review Boards (IRBs) and investigators, in no small part because their requirements appear to constrain the independence of the scientific community.

At the request of the National Institutes of Health (NIH) Office of Research on Women's Health (ORWH), the Institute of Medicine established a Committee on the Ethical and Legal Issues Relating to the Inclusion of Women in Clinical Studies. It is within the context of public doubt about the equitable involvement of women and racial and ethnic groups in clinical research, skepticism about the methods and motives of investigators, and legislation enacted that attempts to address these concerns, that the committee executed its charge.

The committee was asked to examine the ethical and legal implications of policies that seek broader inclusion of women in clinical studies, including pregnant women and women of childbearing potential. In its analysis, the committee was asked to pay particular attention to the participation of women in drug trials and the legal liabilities resulting from injuries to research subjects. The charge did not include a review of the state of scientific knowledge about gender differences, but the committee found that a basic understanding of the subject was necessary to its deliberations.

## WOMEN'S PARTICIPATION IN CLINICAL STUDIES

The current concern about women's participation in clinical studies arises from the conflict of two public policy positions: protectionism and access. Emphasis on the need to protect research subjects burgeoned in the 1950s and 1960s in response to revelations of abuses of the research process. This emphasis was reinforced by the discovery of adverse outcomes in the children of women who had taken certain drugs during pregnancy. In the mid-1970s, legislation was passed that was designed to protect research subjects from unethical treatment. The regulations and guidelines stemming from this legislation also were designed to protect against fetal injury in their restrictions on the inclusion of pregnant women and women of childbearing potential in drug trials.

In recent years, guidelines and regulations put in place to protect research subjects have been challenged by claims that they are overprotective and overly exclusive, and therefore detrimental to the health of the very persons they were intended to protect. This shift in perspective developed in the early and mid-1980s, when women's health groups and Acquired Immune Deficiency Syndrome (AIDS) activists drew attention to inequities in the health research agenda and the exclusion of women and other groups from research studies. Since then, there has been a call for greater access to health care research for women, as well as members of diverse racial and ethnic groups. The shift in emphasis from protectionism to access gained momentum in 1990 with the release of a General Accounting Office (GAO) report that found that NIH had failed to fully implement its 1986 policy of greater inclusion of women in clinical studies, and that women were indeed "underrepresented" in some clinical studies. The report lent credence to the claims that women's health needs were not being adequately addressed and has stimulated legislative efforts to correct the imbalance.

The National Institutes of Health Revitalization Act, passed on June 10, 1993, represents one such effort. The Act includes several provisions relating to clinical studies, one of which has stirred considerable controversy. This much-debated provision requires that each NIH-funded study include representative samples of subpopulations (particularly women and members of diverse racial and ethnic groups) unless their exclusion is justified; notably, cost is not a justifiable criterion for exclusion. The Act is clearly intended to promote justice in clinical research by changing the prevailing assumption of exclusion to one of inclusion, a move strongly supported by many in the research community and by the members of this committee. On the other hand, many—this committee included—have expressed concern that if the act is too rigidly interpreted, it will make costly and unreasonable demands on the scientific research process and impede the implementation of its noble goal.

Before attempting to delineate how the goal of the NIH Revitalization Act might be more effectively achieved, the committee believed it was important to ascertain the current level of women's participation in clinical studies. Are women "underrepresented" in clinical studies, as many have claimed? Like others who had tried to assess women's participation in the whole of clinical research, the committee was frustrated by the lack of any systematic, centralized collection of data on the gender composition of study populations. Although the ORWH has begun such a collection at NIH, the results are not yet available. As an alternative approach, the committee undertook its own data collection and review of the published literature. The committee found the available data inadequate for determining whether women have participated in the whole of clinical studies to the same extent as men, and whether women have been disadvantaged by policies regarding their participation or a failure to focus on their health interests in the conduct of research. The literature detailing past research on heart disease and AIDS does, however, provide some evidence of gender inequity in these areas of study.

The committee can conclude from its survey that there are many unanswered questions about gender-based differences in response to treatment, and that, in general, investigators have not done one or more of the following: reported the results of gender analyses, performed gender analyses of study results, or recruited adequate numbers of women to support the kind of subgroup analysis that would be needed to resolve these questions.

That the committee was unable to draw conclusions about women's participation in clinical research as a whole from available data underscores the need for systematized collection of information. The NIH Revitalization Act's mandate that ORWH create a registry focused solely on women's health and the collection of women's health data is too narrow—without information on men's health issues and men's levels of participation in such studies, monitoring of the relative levels of participation in the future will be difficult and open to bias.

**The committee supports the efforts of NIH to establish a registry of clinical studies and recommends that such a registry include information on the participation of women and men and on the racial and ethnic composition of participants in such studies, as well as the research questions addressed, that such information be reasonably accessible to investigators and the public, and that the scope of the studies included in the registry be comprehensive.**

The committee views this registry as a potentially valuable resource in the development of national research agendas, preparation of reports to Congress, preparation of grant requests by investigators, recruitment of study participants, and development of cooperative efforts among institutes and other study sponsors, including multicenter studies. Such a registry would facilitate the development of the NIH research agenda. Another purpose might be to provide data for reporting to Congress on implementation of the legislative mandate to include women and racial and ethnic groups in clinical studies.

A comprehensive scope is vital to achieving the above purposes and avoiding the potential waste of limited research dollars on duplicative research. At a minimum, the registry should include ongoing studies as well as published studies.

**The committee recommends that NIH work with other federal agencies and departments that conduct clinical research to ensure reporting of all federally funded clinical studies. The committee further recommends that representatives of NIH initiate discussions with FDA concerning the feasibility of including privately funded studies in such a registry.**

The kinds of information to be included and reported to the registry should be uniform. In addition to gender composition of the study population, the registry might include an abstract of the study, the investigator name, and other study population characteristics, such as age and racial and ethnic identification. In implementing such a registry, NIH should consider the costs, reporting pathways, accessibility of information, enforceability of reporting requirements, and quality control. NIH should also consider and take precautions against problems that might be posed by such a registry, particularly with private industry involvement, including considerations of confidentiality, insurance reimbursement implications, endorsement of studies through inclusion in registry, access to non-peer-reviewed studies, administrative burden, and cost considerations.

## JUSTICE IN CLINICAL STUDIES: GUIDING PRINCIPLES

Concerns about justice in the conduct of biomedical research involving human subjects received little attention until the publication in 1978 of the National Commission for the Protection of Human Subjects of Biomedical and Behavioral Research's *Belmont Report*. This report outlined three ethical principles that should govern research: respect for persons, beneficence, and justice. With an understanding that calls to rectify women's alleged "underrepresentation" in clinical studies are based on concerns about unequal distribution of the benefits of biomedical research, the committee chose to form its analysis around principles of justice. Justice is not served when the nation's research agenda ignores important questions regarding the health of one gender when one gender does not participate in clinical studies, and when one gender is treated with interventions that have not been adequately tested in that gender. Based on these observations, the committee recommends three general principles of justice with regard to questions of gender in the conduct of clinical research:

1. **The scientific community and the institutions that support it must ensure that scientific advances in medicine and public health fairly benefit all people, regardless of gender, race, ethnicity, or age. Therefore, the national research agenda must ensure that medical research promotes the health and well-being of both women and men.**

2. **Where it is established that specific health interests of women, men, or other groups have not received a fair allocation of research attention or resources, justice may require a policy of preferential treatment toward these specific areas in order to remedy a past injustice and to avoid perpetuating that injustice.**

3. **Volunteers for clinical studies should be offered the opportunity to participate without regard to gender, race, ethnicity, or age. Women and men should be enrolled as participants in clinical studies in a manner that ensures that research yields scientifically generalizable results applicable to both genders.**

## SCIENTIFIC CONSIDERATIONS

There is a general belief among clinical researchers that, in most situations, women and men will *not* differ significantly in their response to treatment. The evidence to support this belief is not easily assembled, however, and there are countervailing concerns that gender differences have been insufficiently studied. Some of the known gender differences in response to treatments are related to physiological differences between the genders. Important examples include hormonal differences, particularly the variation in drug response by women during different stages of the menstrual cycle, the physiological changes that accompany pregnancy and lactation (conditions that carry the additional concern of the effect of drugs on the fetus and nursing infant), and pharmacokinetic effects such as differential rates of drug absorption and excretion. Hormonal contraceptives and hormone replacement therapy in menopause may also have their own effects on the natural course of disease as well as on diagnosis and treatment interventions. Other differences are psychosocial in origin or are mediated by tendencies of men and women to act differently with respect to health care.

These true gender differences (and differences associated with gender, e.g., weight) have implications for the design of clinical trials, the subset of clinical studies that provides the most rigorous and reliable test of the effectiveness and safety of new drugs and treatment interventions. For example, greater heterogeneity among research subjects may permit the investigator to spot trends that might otherwise be missed, even if the numbers are too small for statistically reliable subgroup analysis. At the same time, greater homogeneity among research subjects reduces unexplained variance.

The committee has focused particularly on treatment trials in reaching its conclusions. The committee finds that the weight of scientific evidence, as well as practical considerations, supports the inclusion of both genders— and indeed all kinds of demographic subgroups—wherever possible. The most compelling scientific reasons for exclusion are found in investigations of diseases, conditions, or risk factors (including behavior) that are highly concentrated in a single gender. Some would argue that excluding women is justified in a study where there is no anticipated difference in how women and men respond to a treatment but where the disease is less common among women. These arguments rest on a false assumption that women's presence diminishes homogeneity and thereby lessens the ability to observe the main effect of the treatment (i.e., whether the treatment is effective for any subject). Person-years of follow-up are person-years of follow-up whether they are female or male years, *unless* the researchers have plausible hypotheses about gender differences in response. And if they *do* have convincing hypotheses about qualitative gender-specific differences, then this too argues for including both genders, but in sufficient numbers to test for gender-specific results.

This is not to say that there are no significant gender-specific diseases or treatment effects, nor does the committee mean to argue that sufficient attention has been paid to the possibility of gender-specific differences. The committee supports the need to examine these issues systematically where they are based on well-grounded scientific hypotheses, and we support attempts to encourage scientists and clinicians to consider and pursue such gender-related hypotheses. The committee acknowledges, however, that most treatments and most diseases do *not* differ significantly by gender. This observation reinforces rather than reduces the justification for a principle of inclusion: if indeed most treatment effects in the setting of treatment trials do not differ by gender, then it is reasonable for treatment trials to include both genders.

In general, the committee's findings are compatible with the goals of NIH's legislative mandate for greater inclusion of women and racial and ethnic groups in clinical studies, albeit with certain important exceptions. When there are no anticipated treatment effects by gender, however, a policy that requires scientists to include sufficient representation of both genders to permit subgroup analyses would require, at a minimum, that clinical studies significantly increase their size (to detect the main effect in each group) and proportionately increase their expenses. In an era of concern about the nation's resources, and about expenditures on health in particular, it is argued that a study-by-study application of this requirement makes for both questionable policy and questionable science. When no subgroup differences are anticipated, *requiring* scientists to enroll sufficient numbers to ensure the statistical power to detect unsuspected differences would produce little additional information at a greatly increased cost. Instead of this blanket requirement, the committee recommends a continuing review of the evidence on gender-specific effects and greater attentiveness to questions of gender at every level of the research process, from the design of individual studies to the setting of the national research agenda.

**The committee recommends that NIH commission a study to identify known gender differences in drug response.**

**The committee recommends that investigators be attentive to factors associated with possible gender differences in drug response and design their studies accordingly. Further, NIH should commission a study that will assist investigators in their effort to detect such differences.**

**The committee recommends that in the design of studies investigators avoid exclusions based on demographic characteristics.**

**The committee recommends that investigators proposing research involving human subjects provide a reasonable review of the evidence and plausibility of gender-specific effects relevant to their research, and that studies be required to be designed with sufficient power to detect subgroup differences only when such a review indicates that such a design is warranted. When there is no information concerning possible gender differences, however, the investigator should, when feasible, include both genders in sufficient number to detect differences.**

Strategies other than clinical trials, (e.g., surveillance techniques) are available to help devise hypotheses about the differential response of men and women to medical interventions. These strategies may be significantly less costly than large-scale clinical trials that include sufficient numbers of men and women to detect gender differences in response.

**The committee recommends that NIH assist investigators in this effort by: (1) identifying, developing, and disseminating alternative methods for detecting or formulating hypotheses about gender differences and (2) providing guidance for the use of these methods by investigators, initial review groups, and study sections.**

## SOCIAL AND ETHICAL CONSIDERATIONS

Clinical research is both shaped and constrained by the social and ethical context in which it takes place. While federal research regulations clearly delineate the ethical boundaries of research involving humans subjects, more subtle social influences—notably, biases—also play a role in determining the diseases and populations that are studied. In a society such as ours, composed of people of different races, ethnicities, and economic backgrounds, both unconscious and conscious biases may render those of lesser status "invisible" (or unimportant) to those of greater power and status. Accordingly, the health interests of persons of lower social status may not receive attention equal to that of the health interests of others. These biases may also operate with respect to gender, where women and their concerns have traditionally been assigned lower status. Two forms of unconscious gender bias have particular relevance for the design and conduct of clinical studies: *male bias* (observer error caused by adopting a male perspective and habit of thought) and the *male norm* (the tendency to use males as the standard and to see females as deviant or problematic, even in studying diseases that affect both sexes). Both have been thought to contribute to a predominant focus on men's health problems and on men as research participants.

Within the scientific community, there is no consensus concerning whether scientific objectivity can be achieved. Some scientists believe that the research process cannot easily be disentangled from the social world within which it is conducted. Societies stratified by gender, race, ethnicity, and socioeconomic status provide different "lenses" through which to see and understand social and scientific reality. These unconscious biases may permeate the entire scientific research process, influencing the research topics selected, the definition and operationalization of concepts examined, the study design, the method of data collection employed, and the research participants chosen for inclusion. Furthermore, such unconscious assumptions contribute to the view that men's physical makeup and experiences are the standard by which to measure and compare women's; to the extent that women's experiences differ from the established male norm, they may be categorized as deviant. These biases impede the progress of the scientific enterprise and produce findings that are not valid for large segments of the population.

**The committee recommends that NIH and IRBs engage in educational efforts that will ensure that investigators are aware of such gender biases and that studies are equitably conceived and designed with respect to gender.**

One way to reduce the influence of such gender biases may be to have a greater number of women scientists active in the research enterprise, through, for example, identification and removal of any institutional barriers to their increased participation. The perspectives they bring to bear may differ markedly from those of their male colleagues, thus aiding in the dissolution of unwarranted and inaccurate assumptions about women in the research enterprise.

**The committee recommends that NIH continue its efforts to encourage women of all racial and ethnic groups to become scientific researchers and to assume positions of authority within the scientific hierarchy.**

Gender is not the only variable that science has been charged with ignoring. There are other important differences among groups—such as race, ethnicity, socioeconomic status—that are capable of affecting health and illness. The lack of attention to or inadequate conceptualization and measurement of these variables in clinical studies has resulted in findings that are inapplicable to particular racial, ethnic, and socioeconomic groups. For example, in order to accurately determine the effects of race on health and treatment outcomes, it is important to clearly distinguish the biological and sociological components of race. Standard methods of data collection may be inappropriate to certain cultural groups and may need to be modified to ensure that the information obtained is valid and for the risk-benefit ratio to be acceptable. Thus, studies must be planned, designed, and executed to produce valid and generalizable results to the populations under investigation. Investigators and IRBs should utilize the expertise of scholars with experience in studying these populations to avoid the weaknesses evidenced in earlier research.

The history of government-sponsored health research and health care efforts in racial, ethnic, and socioeconomic groups has not been unblemished—past unethical treatment has led individuals from these groups to be wary of participation in current studies. Because of the requirements of the NIH Revitalization Act of 1993, researchers now stand to gain or lose support in accordance with their success in recruiting and retaining participants from these same groups, the federal mandate has the potential effect of exacerbating past problems of exploitation. Knowledge of the history of health research in relevant racial or ethnic groups and an awareness of the cultural and political frames of reference employed by the members of these groups will enable researchers to avoid perpetuating the problems.

Informed consent is the primary mechanism for protecting subjects from unethical treatment. NIH, IRBs, and investigators must work together to tailor the consent process so that it will be effective for every group that participates in clinical studies. This entails, for example, both understanding and avoiding what might constitute excessive inducement (monetary or otherwise) for members of a group. If the benefits of research are to accrue to all groups equally, then proper study design and fully informed consent are critical elements to the achievement of that end. Collaboration among clinical investigators, IRBs, and those with research expertise in these groups (e.g., social scientists) would facilitate the design of clinical studies that are socially, as well as scientifically, valid and ethically acceptable.

**The committee recommends that NIH commission a study of attitudinal and institutional barriers to participation in research among women, racial and ethnic groups, and the poor.**

**The committee recommends that NIH train initial review groups (IRGs), technical evaluation groups (TEGs) and investigators in recruitment and retention issues; part of this training should emphasize methodological and ethical issues in conducting research with women of diverse racial and ethnic groups and poor women.**

**The committee recommends that investigators tailor study designs and recruitment and retention efforts to the specific populations to be included in the study. Investigators must consider the relevance of race, ethnicity, socioeconomic status, and other subgroup variables to their study and develop appropriate definitions, methods, and measurements, to ensure the validity of their research efforts among these groups.**

**The committee recommends that in designing recruitment and consent procedures, investigators be cognizant of concerns and needs of communities that have a history of exploitation or abuse in previous clinical studies. Investigators also must ensure that such information be presented and carefully explained, orally and/or in writing, in the potential participant's preferred language.**

## LEGAL CONSIDERATIONS

Health-related research and development in the United States is supported by the federal government (predominantly through the National Institutes of Health [NIH]), the pharmaceutical industry, and private foundations. This institutional structure can affect the conduct of research because it is the source not only of funding, but also of procedures for reviewing the ethics of scientific research—including whether a proposed plan for selecting research participants is just—and of the legal requirements applicable to research.

Current federal policies—in the form of statutes, regulations, and agency guidelines and memoranda—affect the achievement of equity in clinical studies. These policies govern research funded, conducted, or otherwise regulated by the federal government, its agencies, and departments. The policies vary: some appear to promote inclusion of both genders, others refer to inclusion of women and racial and ethnic groups, and others specify conditions applicable to women of childbearing potential and pregnant women. Application of a particular policy may depend on funding origin, type of research, condition studied, or fertility status of the proposed study participant. Particularly in the area of drug development, clinical studies receiving federal funding or performed at institutions supported by federal funding may be subject to a number of policies prior to a drug's entrance into the market. The many recent changes in relevant federal policies promote inclusion, rather than exclusion. As a result, policies have become more congruent. Consistency and, where possible, congruence among these policies is important to promote compliance and prevent confusion.

**The committee recommends that NIH work closely with the FDA and with other Public Health Service (PHS) agencies to make regulations and policies on inclusion of women and racial and ethnic groups consistent with one another and, wherever possible, to make them congruent.**

If the policies of federal agencies are harmonized, there will still remain the task of educating the research community concerning what is required, and motivating that community to comply. Enunciation of sound and congruent policies, in conjunction with a comprehensive educational program, will ensure that policies and the rationales for the policies are properly understood by the research community.

**The committee recommends that NIH, in cooperation with FDA, should institute a comprehensive education program directed at in-**

**vestigators, institutions, and IRBs on policies concerning the inclusion of women and racial and ethnic groups in clinical studies.**

The policies and activities of federal agencies are subject to constitutional challenge and review. It is unclear whether research policies that *constrain* the involvement of women in government-sponsored or government regulated research could be held to violate constitutional standards of liberty and equality. Such challenges could possibly be based in principles of decisional privacy and equal protection derived from the Fourteenth Amendment. For example, the Fourteenth Amendment's protection of "life, liberty, and property" has been interpreted to provide decisional privacy with respect to terminating life-sustaining treatment and obtaining an abortion. It remains to be seen, however, how this protection could be read to imply a right to assume the risk of taking an experimental drug. Similarly, the Fourteenth Amendment guarantees all citizens "equal protection of the laws," which the Supreme Court has interpreted as prohibiting the government from treating similar individuals and groups differently. Research policies that result in the exclusion of women as a class might be found to contradict the equal protection clause unless a court found the justification for such exclusion to be adequate.

Both individuals and organizations involved in the conduct of research must deal with another set of legal considerations—liability. Fear of potential legal liability has been cited as one of the reasons that women of childbearing age and pregnant women have traditionally been excluded from clinical trials of drugs. The focus of liability concerns is on possible injury to potential offspring. Although recent evidence may indicate that exposure of a father to some chemicals may cause harm to a developing fetus, the focus has overwhelmingly been on the potential for harm to offspring resulting from the mother's exposure either before or after conception.

More recently, pharmaceutical companies have begun to recognize that they could also be liable for *not* including women in clinical research. For example, a pharmaceutical company may be liable if a drug that has never been tested in women is nevertheless marketed for use by both genders and prescribed for a woman who then suffers an adverse reaction. Similar approaches to liability could be used as well where men, or subpopulations of women or men, were not included in a study population but suffered an injury. This creates a paradox for clinical trial sponsors whose efforts to exclude women in order to protect themselves from liability may actually risk liability for exclusion.

The committee concluded that it is impossible to quantify the risk of tort liability from the inclusion of women in clinical studies at this time, because: (1) there is no complete compendium of *unreported* cases involving settlements and (2) pregnant women and women of childbearing age have not been included in some major studies in the past. But, difficulties of prediction are compounded even more because tort law is governed by the individual states, with many variations on issues such as whether a woman's informed consent will serve to bar an independent action by a child injured as a fetus during such research. Analysis of existing legal rules and principles seems to indicate that the likelihood of successful damage actions is limited. Nevertheless, broadening the research population to include those groups previously excluded may also generate additional legal actions that will test existing legal doctrine.

Although there is a general lack of case law on liability for injuries to research participants, there is some precedent for liability for exclusion from research. The case law suggests that if a drug was found to cause injuries to women, and yet women had been excluded from clinical trials of the drug, the sponsor might be held liable for failing to test the drug in women. For some drugs, however, the potential for teratogenic or mutagenic effects is low or the negative effects are manifested after a long latent period. For these drugs, even adequate testing in all relevant populations unfortunately may not reveal their potential to cause harm.

The committee recognizes that, regardless of their basis or justification, fears about liability are real. On balance, however, the committee concludes that liability concerns should not represent an impediment to implementation of public policies that favor the broader inclusion of women in clinical studies.

A special set of concerns in the research area stems from the differing bases for liability according to which party is a defendant. A pharmaceutical company, for example, might be sued on the basis of strict liability, while a researcher ordinarily would be sued only on the basis of negligence in the informed consent process. With regard to the latter, the new federal policies calling for inclusion of women in clinical studies will help establish new standards that will be relevant to legal actions.

Many of the concerns voiced about liability in the context of research including women are the same as those with regard to the tort system in general. For example, expert scientific testimony is necessary to establish that a particular drug caused an injury. There are inherent difficulties in assuring the unbiased nature of such testimony in what are often highly technical cases.

**The committee recommends that current and future initiatives toward general tort reform include attention to issues of research-related injury, including issues of proof of causation.**

The question of whether there should be a special compensation scheme for injuries sustained by children as a result of a parent's participation in a clinical study is similar to that raised in the context of research subjects in general. Because of the difficulty in quantifying the risk of liability, the committee does not recommend adoption—at this time—of a special compensation scheme limited to coverage of children injured prenatally or preconceptually. Any new compensation scheme focusing only on such injuries poses especially difficult problems with regard to establishing causation and averting large numbers of questionable recoveries.

**The committee recommends that NIH thoroughly review the area of compensation for research injury in general and that consideration of implementation of any compensation scheme include attention to prenatal and preconceptual injuries to children resulting from a parent's participation in a clinical study.**

Our current health care reimbursement system does not include coverage for medical care resulting from injuries sustained during research. This could be accomplished through a system of universal access with adequate coverage.

**The committee recommends that health care reform efforts include considerations of medical care for research-related injury.**

## RISKS TO REPRODUCTION AND OFFSPRING

Historically, concern for the risks of new drugs has focused on women of reproductive potential, including pregnant and lactating women, but risks to the male reproductive system also may merit attention. Men and women of reproductive age get sick and take medications, and drugs intended for use by this population should therefore be tested in this population. Some of these drugs, however, have potential risks to reproduction or for the development of offspring. These risks give added importance to informed consent and contraceptive options. Risk assessment for reproductive and developmental toxicity may be complicated by the high background rates of infertility and birth defects, as well as the difficulty of identifying the specific effects of the drug under investigation. Techniques, such as animal studies, in vitro analysis, as well as surveillance for developmental effects, among others, can provide some information on potential hazards to humans. Laboratory animals and humans can differ in toxicokinetics, however, and the use of data from animals to determine health risks in humans must be assessed carefully.

Investigators should take these reproductive and developmental risks into consideration in the design and conduct of clinical trials. If men and women of reproductive potential are included in a trial in which they will be exposed to a potential reproductive or developmental toxicant, the potential risks must be characterized as accurately as possible so they can make an informed decision about whether or not to participate. If they decide to participate, they also may wish to consider measures to prevent pregnancy. Information about toxicity risk can help participants determine the likelihood that the baseline incidence of adverse pregnancy outcomes will have been increased by study participation, should a pregnancy occur during the trial. When the study involves lactating women, the exposure and impact of the agent on the nursing infant also should be discussed.

**The committee recommends that investigators and IRBs not exclude persons of reproductive age from participation in clinical studies. In the case of women of reproductive age, the potential or prospect of becoming pregnant during the study may not be used as a justification for precluding or limiting participation. Risks to the reproductive system should be considered in the same manner as risks to other organ systems. Risks to possible offspring of both men and women who are not pregnant or lactating should not be considered in the risk-benefit calculation. It is the responsibility of investigators and IRBs to assure that the informed consent process includes an adequate discussion of risks to reproduction and potential offspring, including, where appropriate, an adequate discussion of relevant considerations of birth control.**

**The committee recommends that the participant be permitted to select voluntarily the contraceptive method of his or her choice where there are no relevant study-dependent, scientific reasons for excluding certain contraceptives (e.g., drug interaction).**

**The committee recommends that pregnancy termination options be discussed as part of the consent process in clinical studies that pose unknown or foreseeable risks to potential offspring.**

**The committee recommends that investigators and IRBs not exclude women who are lactating from participation in clinical studies. It is the responsibility of investigators and IRBs to ensure that the informed consent process includes, wherever appropriate, an advisory to potential participants that there may be special risks to their children if nursing mothers participate. No nursing mother should be permitted to agree to participate without first receiving additional information about these special risks.**

The inclusion of pregnant women in clinical studies, creates new concerns and risks, but the lack of proven safe treatment options for ill pregnant women carries its own set of concerns and risks. The committee believes that it is important to encourage clinical research to advance the medical management of pregnant women who are or may become ill.

**The committee recommends that NIH strongly encourage and facilitate clinical research to advance the medical management of pre-existing medical conditions in women who become pregnant (e.g., lupus), medical conditions of pregnancy (e.g., gestational diabetes) and, conditions that threaten the successful course of pregnancy (e.g., pre-term labor).**

Clinical trials (as well as other studies) have limited power to detect some adverse effects due to the relatively small numbers of subjects included in research compared with the number of persons who eventually may use the drug under study. Adverse effects may not become evident until the drug is in widespread use. Therefore, systematic surveillance for developmental effects is essential to any plan to include pregnant women in clinical research. Together, both methods will further our understanding of the medical management of the ill pregnant woman.

**The committee recommends that a review be undertaken of existing birth defects monitoring programs to critically define what they are capable of doing and suggest improvements and reasonable expectations for their use.**

In the context of encouraging clinical research to advance the medical management of pregnant women who are or may become ill, the committee reviewed the current Department of Health and Human Services (DHHS) regulations concerning the involvement of pregnant women as research subjects. The committee's review of current DHHS regulations was limited to situations in which the pregnant woman is the subject of the research. It did *not* include situations involving fetal research (currently covered by the same regulation) since this topic was outside of the committee's charge.

The DHHS regulations begin with a presumption of exclusion—that is, "no pregnant woman may be a research subject" except under certain conditions; the regulations also classify pregnant women as a "vulnerable population" deserving of special protection. In this context, "vulnerable" suggests that pregnant women are less autonomous or more easily exploited, by virtue of their pregnancy, than other persons—an inference that the committee has found no evidence to support. Removal of pregnant women from the regulatory category of "vulnerable" potential subjects would avoid any such inference.

The committee was unanimous in the view that pregnant women should be presumed to be eligible for participation in clinical studies. The committee also unanimously endorsed the importance of recognizing in public policy as well as in the deliberations of IRBs and investigators, that pregnant women should be treated as competent adults capable of making their own decisions about participation in research.

**The committee recommends that pregnant women be presumed to be eligible for participation in clinical studies. It is the responsibility of investigators and IRBs to ensure that pregnant women are provided with adequate information about the risks and benefits to themselves, their pregnancies and their potential offspring. Even when evidence concerning risks is unknown or ambiguous, the decision about acceptability of risk to the pregnancy or to offspring should be made by the woman as part of the informed consent process.**

It is critical to note that the committee *is not* advocating active recruitment of pregnant women into each and every clinical study. Rather, it is urging that the prevailing presumption regarding the participation of pregnant women in clinical trials and other intervention studies be shifted from one of *exclusion* to one of *inclusion*. The committee believes that a strengthened informed consent process can address specific concerns regarding the inclusion of pregnant women in clinical studies. This process should include a special disclosure statement detailing in lay language what is known about the risks and benefits of participation. The statement should be reviewed carefully with the pregnant woman and she should be encouraged to consult with her obstetrical care provider as well as with the potential baby's father. Only after the woman demonstrates an adequate understanding of the risks and benefits of participation should consent be solicited. It should be noted that the committee rejects any requirement that the consent of the potential baby's father be a condition of the participation of a pregnant woman in research.

The committee recognizes that, as in all clinical studies, there may be scientifically and medically valid reasons for excluding pregnant women from a particular study. A pregnant woman would be excluded if the medical condition of pregnancy disqualifies her as a subject in the same sense that anyone else, pregnant or nonpregnant, would be disqualified based on medical conditions that would interfere scientifically with the study. For example, a pregnant woman would be excluded from a study of hormone replacement or contraception.

Recording by the IRB in writing of both its reasons for permitting any exception to the general presumption of inclusion of pregnant women and frequency with which it grants such exceptions would help the IRBs to implement properly any exceptions to the presumption. There was considerable discussion within the committee about whether there are any exceptional instances in which IRBs can be given the discretion to exclude pregnant women from participation for other than scientific reasons. *Most* committee members ultimately endorsed the following recommendation:

> **Investigators and IRBs may exclude pregnant women from participation only when the IRB finds, and records its finding in writing, that the following standard has been met: (1) there is no prospect of medical benefit to the pregnant woman, and (2) a risk of significant harm to potential offspring is known or can be plausibly inferred.**

A finding that a risk of significant harm to potential offspring is "known or can be plausibly inferred" may be based on evidence from animal studies, in vitro studies, structure-activity relationship data, or previous clinical experience. Under the above standard, IRBs may exclude pregnant women from the earliest phases of many drug trials, but most clinical studies would remain open to pregnant women.

A few members of the committee, however, were not able to endorse the above standard. They wished to reserve for the IRB the discretion to exclude pregnant women from participation not only when there is no prospect of medical benefit to the women but also when there is the potential for benefit to them that could be characterized as minimal or insignificant.

The committee also struggled with how to accommodate within its support for the shift of the presumption to *inclusion* of pregnant women (from that of exclusion) a role for conscience and an individual investigator's moral commitments. It was agreed that, at a minimum, such a mechanism would require that the investigator provide the IRB with a written explanation of his or her concerns of conscience and that the IRB review any such requests in light of a presumption that favors the inclusion of pregnant women in clinical studies. It is because of the potential for abuse of a "conscience" exemption that the committee could not resolve whether or under what conditions such an exemption should be constructed.

At least a technical amendment to Subpart A, sec. 46.111(a)(3), eliminating the reference to pregnant women as a "vulnerable population" will be required by the recommended revision to Subpart B.

> **The committee recommends that OPRR revise and reissue subpart B of the DHHS regulations for the Protection of Human Subjects, titled "Additional Protections Pertaining to Research, Development, and Related Activities Involving Fetuses, Pregnant Women, and Human**

**In-vitro Fertilization [45 C.F.R. 46, subpart B] in accordance with the committee's recommendation.**

## IMPLEMENTATION

Policies requiring the inclusion of women and racial and ethnic groups in clinical studies are already in place. The present emphasis placed by NIH on the recruitment of diverse population groups into clinical research is a strong initial step in the pursuit of equity in clinical studies. Where earlier versions of the current NIH policy on inclusion of women in clinical studies simply encouraged investigators to include women in study populations, more recent policy statements require that "clear and compelling" rationales be given for the exclusion of women from proposed research. The challenge for those involved in clinical research is to achieve full implementation of these guidelines in a way that enhances the overall enterprise *and* deals with the various problems identified by this report. The committee believes that every level of the research structure must actively participate in the efforts to increase subgroup participation in clinical studies. However, the committee does not believe that the interests of justice in advancing the health of all people are best served by an exceptionless requirement that *every* clinical study be large enough to conduct valid analyses of every relevant subgroup comparison. As reflected in the committee's guiding principles 1 and 2 (see Chapter 3), the final burden for achieving justice falls on the national research agenda as a whole and cannot be implemented by a mechanical approach to the selection of subjects on a study-by-study basis.

The ultimate criteria for judging the success of a public policy to achieve justice and promote inclusion will be changes in research policy and clinical practice, and ultimately improvements in health status indicators, particularly in areas where unjustifiable disparities currently exist. Specific objectives include the following:

- Establish accountability for implementation at every level of the research enterprise, including levels well above that of the individual investigator;
- Provide the necessary database to shape adherence and identify gaps in knowledge;
- Establish a system for monitoring compliance with specific inclusion-based requirements and evaluating the extent to which fairness is being achieved;
- Use the preceding processes and data bases to educate, inform, and promote discussion among policy makers, bureaucrats, investigators, IRBs, IRGs, TEGs, and the general public.

The committee has attempted to frame its recommendations as actions that can be taken by all of the actors in the research process, some immediately and some in the longer term, to ensure the broad participation of women and other groups in clinical studies and to advance fairly the health of all persons. The committee strongly believes that tracking both the study populations' composition and topics of funded studies, and providing this information on a regular basis to all those involved in the research process, will in and of itself raise the level of awareness and activity concerning the issues of both study composition and attention to women's health concerns.

## The Investigator

### Immediate Actions

NIH already requires investigators to report the composition of study populations, which keeps investigators aware of the need to involve diverse populations. It is important that individual investigators be aware of both the state of the science and the state of clinical practice with respect to gender and other subgroup differences in their areas of research. **In designing studies, investigators should conduct literature reviews to determine (1) the extent to which an evidentiary base exists for suspecting gender-specific and subgroup effect, and (2) the extent to which women and other groups have served as participants in relevantly similar research.**

**If there is a plausible basis for suspecting gender differences, investigators should make every effort to recruit sufficient participants of both genders to conduct analyses to detect these differences. In the absence of such an evidentiary base, investigators should recruit participants of both genders. Where sample size is large enough, investigators also should conduct analysis of gender differences in these studies.** Investigators should strive to collect sufficient data on gender-related variables to permit a refined interpretation of any observed gender differences (e.g., potential confounders or mechanistic variables such as hormonal status of women, weight, and adiposity) and to reveal trends or suggest hypotheses.

### As Soon as Feasible

**Investigators should draw on the expertise available in the social science community to improve the ways in which the variables of gender, race, and ethnicity are conceptualized, operationalized and measured in their studies.** Such collegial exchanges will enable investigators to tailor their study designs, recruitment and retention efforts, and informed consent procedures to the study population selected, to avoid unwarranted exclusions of potential participants, and to be prepared to collect sufficient data on gender-related and subgroup variables to analyze for confounding effects.

Investigators clearly need broad-based support from the other actors within the research process in order to carry out their part of a comprehensive agenda. **The committee recommends that IRBs, IRGs, TEGs, scientific advisory councils, and NIH management become more directly involved with investigators in activities that promote development of more inclusive study designs.** Measures recommended by the committee, such as IRB review of protocols for study population composition and NIH provision of opportunities for investigator training and access to needed databases, facilitate investigator efforts to realize the goal of greater inclusion.

## The IRB

### Immediate Actions

**As part of the IRBs' responsibility for ensuring the just selection of persons to be participants in research, IRBs should require investigators to provide the proposed gender, racial, and ethnic composition for each study, as well as information about the distribution of the condition under study in the population at large and the composition of subjects in previous relevant research. It is the IRBs' responsibility to make a determination that the composition of the proposed study is equitable.**

### As Soon as Feasible

**IRBs, in concert with NIH, should engage in educational efforts that will ensure awareness among investigators of gender and racial and ethnic biases.** Research organizations could draw upon the expertise of social scientists experienced in the conceptualization, operationalization, measurement, and analysis of variables relevant to these issues to assist investigators.

The committee believes that providing feedback to IRBs concerning the characteristics of the study populations and research topics it has approved will serve to raise the level of awareness of IRBs to issues of justice and inclusion. **The NIH Office of Protection from Research Risks (OPRR) should require IRBs to collect data on study population composition and research topics of all studies subject to IRB review.** OPRR could monitor study population composition through, for example, a representative sample of general assurance IRBs.

## IRGs and TEGs

### Immediate Actions

Once NIH policies for inclusion of gender, racial, and ethnic groups are finalized, it is anticipated that IRGs and TEGs will have significant responsibility for monitoring their implementation. As with any new policy, it is expected that in the initial stages of implementation guidance will be needed. **NIH should develop a mechanism for monitoring the actions taken by IRGs and TEGs in implementing policies for inclusion of gender, racial, and ethnic groups, and provide feedback to the IRGs and TEGs in order to ensure consistent and appropriate interpretation of these policies.** Among other tools for evaluation, NIH might consider taking a random sample of justifications for exclusions. Central review and evaluation can standardize the implementation of the policy, and it will correct both unnecessarily strict and overly lenient policy interpretations by the peer review system. It will also provide illustrative material for education of IRG and TEG members as recommended below.

### As Soon as Feasible

**Each IRG and TEG should recruit members with expertise in the area of gender, racial, and ethnic differences or persons sensitive to gender and racial and ethnic concerns. Furthermore, every member of IRGs and TEGs should receive training and education on evaluation of study population composition and gender, racial, and ethnic differences.** The very presence of qualified males and females from different racial and ethnic backgrounds is one way of increasing the likelihood that the relevant questions and appropriate conceptualizations are considered by investigators. A rough measure of sensitivity could be based on professional activities, such as research agenda, participation in committees of professional associations, publications, and service at one's institution.

## Scientific Advisory Councils

### As Soon as Feasible

**Mechanisms should be developed for ensuring that principles of justice are central considerations in the setting of the nation's research agenda.** Because clinical research carries both benefits and burdens, justice requires that no one group—gender, racial, ethnic, or socioeconomic—receive disproportionate benefits or bear disproportionate burdens of research. For the overall biomedical research agenda to comply with the requirements of justice, studies must not only include women as well as men, but also women and men from different age cohorts and different racial and ethnic groups. In addition, the health needs of all women and men should receive their fair share of research resources and attention. Scientific advisory councils have the ultimate responsibility for determining priorities in the research agenda for the subject matter area they cover. These decisions should move toward establishing equity in U.S. research efforts for all populations over time. Databases compiled by NIH can be used by scientific advisory councils in making decisions about research priorities within the available funding and in determining what areas require requests for proposals (RFPs) or requests for applications (RFAs) to improve the balance of research across diseases and subgroups. The heads of the councils should confer periodically to assess the application of principles of justice across research areas. In developing research priorities, these councils should give special consideration as to whether the health needs of pregnant women are being adequately addressed by their institutes.

## NIH

**Immediate Actions**

**NIH should maintain the current policy emphasis on the inclusion of women in NIH-supported clinical studies.** NIH should continue the practice of identifying research concerns of various subgroups (gender, race, ethnicity, socioeconomic status) and offer RFAs and RFPs for such studies. **Where new requirements for subgroup analysis result in increases in study size and additional recruitment strategies, supplemental funds (e.g., from the NIH Office of Research on Women's Health) should be made available to meet these funding challenges.**

**NIH should commission studies to determine the present state of scientific knowledge on gender, racial, and ethnic differences to help investigators determine where subgroup analysis would be likely to identify clinically significant differences.** These efforts should culminate in the establishment of a database that includes such information as differences in disease incidence and prevalence, as well as relevant physiological and cultural differences in subgroups. Investigators would be able to consult this database in developing strategies to identify and detect gender, racial, and ethnic differences.

**NIH should require that proposals for clinical studies include in their literature reviews the following: the extent to which an evidentiary base exists for suspecting gender or other subgroup differences relevant to the proposed research; the demographic characteristics of subjects in past similar research; groups for which the proposed study might have**

special relevance; how the preceding information justifies the population selected for the proposed study; and how that choice will address
gaps identified in the literature. This requirement should be incorporated
into the guidelines on the grant application (PHS 398 form).

NIH should widely disseminate to the scientific community methodological guidance on: (1) compliance with the legislative mandate regarding the inclusion of women and other subgroups in clinical research and (2) considerations for valid subgroup analysis.

## As Soon as Feasible

NIH should pursue the current dialogue with Congress and the research community on the policy of inclusion and the commitment to
justice. The objective is to develop mechanisms that merge public policy
goals with scientific advice to promote legislation that is at once socially
responsible, practical, and consistent with good science. Such action would
extract the scientific community from a current dilemma: if NIH is strictly
responsive to the law, clinical studies may become larger and more expensive in order to be in compliance, with no guarantee that this is either the
most efficient or effective way to advance the health interests of women or
other groups. If this results in an inability to fund an adequate range of
biomedical research, it is likely that the health interests of all people will
suffer, and thus justice will not be served.

As part of the registry of clinical studies it is currently evaluating, NIH
should establish a database cross-referenced by: (1) categories of disease
and physiological or psychological factors and (2) study population composition of ongoing and published studies. This database should be compiled
in a way that ensures easy accessibility to the data included by subgroup
classification. Reporting requirements for all studies should be comprehensive and uniform and at a minimum include: the research questions addressed and the gender, race, ethnicity, socioeconomic status, age, and hormonal status (i.e., pregnancy, stage of menstrual cycle) of the study population.

To facilitate the collection of data about inclusion and justice from
non-federally supported research, NIH should encourage journal publishers to require presentation of data on demographic characteristics.
Currently, there is no national norm that compels pharmaceutical manufacturers and other investigators to submit their data to a registry or other data
repository.

NIH should assist investigators in the effort to detect gender differences by: (1) identifying, developing, and disseminating alternative methods
for detecting or formulating hypotheses about gender differences and
(2) providing guidance for the use of these methods by investigators,
IRGs, and TEGs. The new legislative mandate makes it especially critical

that both investigators and review committees clearly understand the inter-relationship of sample sizes and the power to draw statistically significant inferences about differences between subgroups. A proactive strategy of development and dissemination would help investigators in complying with regulations. It would also help to prevent the introduction into the literature of analyses based on insufficient data—analyses that could ultimately do a disservice to subgroups by fostering seemingly valid but erroneous conclusions.

# 1

# Introduction

In response to the frequent claims that women's health has been less well served than men's health by clinical research practices and policies, the scientific community has begun to devote increased attention to what has now become a central public policy concern. It is contended that women are participants in clinical studies less frequently than men and that this affects the study of women's health in two central ways: (1) women's experiences and manifestations of health problems common to both men and women are not addressed; and, (2) health conditions specific to women (e.g., menopause) are not adequately investigated. In the past three years, both the National Institutes of Health (NIH) and Food and Drug Administration (FDA), two pivotal players in the biomedical research process, have issued new policies that are changing the ways women are studied by the research community. In June, Congress passed the NIH Revitalization Act of 1993 (P.L. 103-43), which mandates the increased inclusion of women and racial and ethnic groups in clinical studies. Several other bills concerning this issue are currently pending before Congress.

In order to responsibly and effectively respond to these concerns and initiatives, the research community must examine the available empirical evidence; determine the nature, scope, and severity of the problem; and then recommend action based on this assessment. A comprehensive analysis of the problems also requires the identification of criteria or standards for judging the proper balance of involvement of women and men, and their interests, in research. This report attempts to identify and elaborate the factors that must be part of systematic examination of such criteria.

## MANDATE AND SCOPE OF STUDY

At the request of the NIH Office of Research on Women's Health, the Institute of Medicine established a Committee on the Ethical and Legal Issues Relating to the Inclusion of Women in Clinical Studies. The committee's report is intended to provide guidance to NIH and to institutional review boards, scientists, and others who design and monitor clinical studies regarding appropriate policies for the admission of women to these studies.

This committee was asked to examine only the ethical and legal issues related to the participation of women as participants in clinical studies. In its attempt to execute this charge, however, the committee found it necessary to look at the accumulated scientific evidence and prevailing methods of clinical investigation in order to understand the principles behind the design of clinical studies and the relevance of biological and physiological differences between the sexes. Without this foundation of understanding, the committee believed it could not build reasoned ethical and legal arguments to support recommendations concerning future research policy.

## STRUCTURE OF REPORT

This report was prompted by concerns that there has been insufficient attention in biomedical research to women's health conditions, and that studies of conditions affecting both genders may not be generalizable to women if they rely primarily on male participants. Chapter 2 provides a brief review of the history and current status of clinical research on women and attempts to gauge current levels of participation. The issues raised by these concerns are complex and controversial, involving considerations of ethics, science, and law, all of which may pose potential constraints on the participation by women in clinical studies.

First, there are compelling ethical arguments for the involvement of women and women's health interests in clinical research. Principles of justice require that all people and social groups be treated fairly. In the context of research, fair treatment requires that men and women be allowed to share equally in both the burdens and benefits of participation in research. Chapter 3 examines these ethical arguments and develops the basic principles that will guide the rest of the report.

Second, an overreliance upon male participants in clinical studies may also make for bad science. Chapter 4 examines some of the known biological, behavioral, and social differences between the genders. These differences are real and significant, and they can affect responses to drugs and other treatments, creating the potential for differential health outcomes based on these documented differences. Consequently, it is not clear that results obtained from male-only studies can always be reliably and safely generalized to female populations. This uncertainty has practical ramifications for clinicians, who may not be able to recommend therapies and prescribe drugs to women when the only data available for decisions are derived from men.

Third, the social and historical context within which research occurs exerts powerful and often hidden influences on the scientific process. Chapter 5 examines the biases that permeate society and may distort the vision of the scientific community, leading to unjust treatment of gender, racial, and ethnic groups.

Fourth, there are concerns about the legal implications of including women in clinical studies—or of excluding them. For example, researchers focus on the potential for harm to the offspring of participants. At the same time, drug manufacturers may be subject to liability if a drug causes injury in a population on which it has *not* been tested. Chapter 6 examines these concerns in detail.

All these concerns are heightened with regard to the participation of women in early-stage drug trials and the risks those trials may pose to reproduction and fetal development. The drug development process is described in a later section of this introduction. Chapter 7 examines the scientific, social, ethical, and legal issues raised by these risks to reproduction and offspring.

Finally, based on full consideration of all these factors, the committee makes specific recommendations for the fair and effective inclusion of women and women's health interests in clinical research. While these recommendations address legal and ethical issues, they necessarily involve scientific and social considerations as well. Chapter 8 also provides direct, practical guidance to NIH with regard to implementing its recommendations.

## DEFINITIONS

In the process of its deliberations, the committee endeavored to be careful with terminology that might be vague or inappropriately value laden. A few definitional clarifications and "sensitive" words are discussed below.

*Women* in this report refers to all females of all racial, ethnic, and socioeconomic backgrounds throughout the adult life cycle, including pregnant and lactating women. Unless otherwise specified, the report addresses the issues in relation to women as a class or to identified subgroups of women, and not women as individuals. Where appropriate, however, the report distinguishes between such class or subgroup interests and individual interests (for example, when discussing the risks and benefits of participating in a particular study).

Our report construes the term *clinical studies* broadly. The definition includes studies that require the involvement of human subjects, as well as studies that review records or data already in existence, but excludes research on animals. Clinical studies include randomized clinical trials of treatments and preventive interventions, as well as observational, behavioral, psychosocial, and medical outcomes studies. The committee acknowledges that some of the more complex ethical and legal issues arise in the context of clinical trials of drugs, and the report distinguishes such trials from other studies when appropriate (see below and Chapter 4).

Two imprecise terms have been widely employed to refer to the perceived lower rates of participation by women in clinical studies: *underrepresentation* and *exclusion*. The report endeavors to limit the use of these terms, which have multiple meanings and thus are often unclear. *Underrepresentation,* for example, has been claimed both: (1) when the proportion of female (or male) participants is less than the proportion of females (or males) affected by the disease under study and (2) when the study design provides inadequate statistical power to detect gender differences. Underrepresentation can also include studies or situations in which men and women are included in proportion to their numbers in the population that experiences the disease, and in sufficient numbers to support statistically valid subgroup analyses, but such analyses are not done.

In contrast, the term *exclusion* is generally understood to apply when women (or men) are explicitly barred from participation because of an express stipulation in the study protocol. In reported study findings, however, it is often difficult to distinguish between explicit exclusion and the failure or inability to recruit sufficient participants or conduct adequate analysis. And regardless of how the terms *underrepresentation* and *exclusion* are expressed or understood, they fail to capture broader considerations that are also critical to this report, such as the failure to adequately address women's (or men's) health issues in the overall research agenda or the failure to investigate outcomes or processes of particular interest to one gender when that gender is included in a study population.

It is also useful to distinguish between *sex* and *gender.* In general, the term *sex* refers to physiological and anatomical differences between men and women. *Gender* refers to the entire set of behaviors and social roles common to a particular sex in a given society. In the interest of consistency, the committee chose to use one term when referring to both men and women, selecting *gender* for use throughout this report.

## THE DRUG DEVELOPMENT PROCESS

Much of the concern that led to this study has centered on drug trials, particularly the timing of the exposure of fertile women to experimental drugs that may do harm to fertility, pregnancy, and fetal development. (See Box 1-1 for a description of the drug development and approval process.) There is usually a substantial body of knowledge about both the disease being treated and the drug being tested by the time a drug enters clinical investigation (see Figure 1-1). For many diseases, the natural history may be reasonably well understood—knowledge of the natural history of a disease is essential to an understanding of whether an intervention (whether pharmaceutical, surgical, or other procedure) is likely to have a beneficial impact. Political factors, however, may modify the typical process of drug development. For example, some drugs thought to be effective in treating human immunodeficiency virus (HIV) may have an accelerated timeline for testing in humans.

For diseases for which beneficial drug therapies exist, there is also likely to be some understanding of how the drugs act to modify the progression or etiology of the disease. This knowledge can be used to suggest modifications in the structure of new drugs, alterations in the treatment schedule (timing or dosing, for example, with meals) for existing drugs, or realization of the potential value of existing drugs not previously used in the treatment of the disease.

By the time a new drug is available for testing in humans, a substantial body of information has already been collected. For example, the chemical will have been evaluated for its ability to alter the etiology and progression of the disease from both in vivo and in vitro testing systems. At the same time, additional data are being gathered concerning the drug's most likely side effects and toxicities. Methods for collecting such data include a series of tests in animals, which may range from days to months in length and involve additional reproductive and offspring studies. Examples of endpoints of these animal testing requirements are displayed in Table 1-1. In vitro testing is also performed to evaluate the potential mechanisms of toxicity and side effects.

These data are then gathered and used to evaluate the potential efficacy of the drug, as well as its likely side effects and toxicity. This information is almost always available before any generalized clinical testing is done in humans. The two exceptions are the completion of the second-generation animal reproductive exposure studies, which generally are not completed until the middle of Phase II (primary efficacy and safety human tests), and chronic toxicity (predominantly conducted to determine carcinogenicity). These studies, which require two years of testing in two animal species, often are not started until Phase II and are not completed until shortly before the filing of a New Drug Application (NDA).

If, after all of these evaluation activities, the drug's potential for benefit in treating disease appears to be greater than its side effects and toxicity, a clinical trial program is developed. Over the course of a clinical trial, atten-

## BOX 1-1 THE DRUG DEVELOPMENT AND APPROVAL PROCESS

It takes 12 years on average for an experimental drug to travel from lab to medicine chest. Only five in 5,000 compounds that enter preclinical testing make it to human testing. One of these five tested in people is approved.

| | Preclinical Testing | Clinical Trials Phase I | Clinical Trials Phase II | Clinical Trials Phase III | FDA | Phase IV |
|---|---|---|---|---|---|---|
| **Years** | 3.5 | 1 | 2 | 3 | 2.5 | **12 Total** |
| **Test Popula-tion** | Laboratory and animal studies | 20 to 80 healthy volunteers | 100 to 300 patient volunteers | 1,000 to 3,000 patient volunteers | | |
| **Purpose** | Assess safety and biological activity | Determine safety and dosage | Evaluate effectiveness, look for side effects. | Verify effectiveness, monitor adverse reactions from long-term use. | Review process/ approval | Additional post-marketing testing required by FDA |
| **Success Rate** | 5,000 compounds evaluated | | 5 enter trials | | 1 approved | |

FILE IND AT FDA     FILE NDA AT FDA

SOURCE: Wierenga and Eaton (1993).

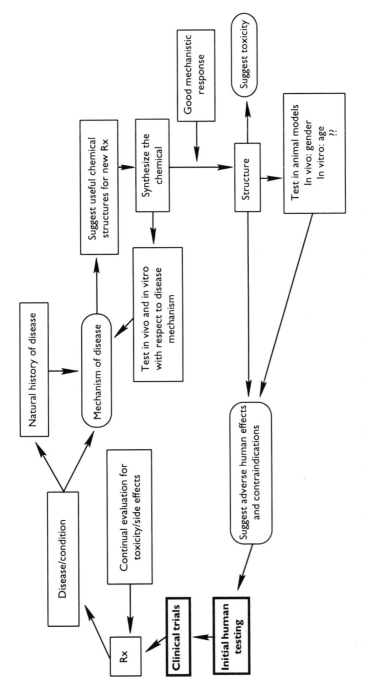

**FIGURE 1-1** Where does a clinical trial stand in the pathway of knowledge development?

TABLE 1-1   Examples of End Points for Various Toxicity Studies

| Study | Endpoints |
| --- | --- |
| Developmental toxicity | Fetus: mortality, growth retardation, skeletal variations, gross external malformations, soft tissue/internal organ defects |
| | Female parent: general toxicity |
| Reproductive toxicity | Male parent: general toxicity, effects on fertility, reproductive organ changes |
| | Offspring: effects on viability, sex ratio, growth, behavior |
| Carcinogenicity | Tumor development and general toxicity |
| Neurotoxicity | Behavior, function, and motor activity deficits; microscopic nervous tissue changes |
| Mutagenicity | Heritable lesions leading to altered phenotypes |

SOURCE: EPA, 1984.

tion is directed toward the identification of dosage range, toxicity, and side effects in treated individuals compared with individuals who receive a standard drug or a placebo, as well as the drug's benefit in treating the disease.

Because animal testing may not identify all types of human toxicity, initial testing of the drug in humans is generally performed under close observation in a series of trials (see Box 1-1). The initial clinical trials (Phase I) are conducted primarily to determine appropriate adult human dosage. Factors evaluated during these initial clinical trials include rate and extent of absorption by the routes chosen for administration. These tests generally can be conducted on a small number of healthy volunteers, although in some instances the testing may be conducted on individuals with the disease targeted for treatment. In Phase II clinical trials, the safety and efficacy of the drug is studied in a small number (on the order of 100) of individuals and the effectiveness of the drug in treating the disease (or diseases) is evaluated; the initial evaluation of toxicity, side effects, and contraindications is extended. It is not uncommon in practice for Phase I and Phase II to be combined.

If the effectiveness of the drug still appears promising and observed side effects and toxicity acceptable, it is studied in a larger number of patients (Phase III). During this phase, several thousand individuals with the appropriate diseases are studied during treatment to verify effectiveness, toxicity, and side effects. If a drug has progressed through all three initial phases of clinical trials and appears to have therapeutic benefit, all of the collected data are gathered, summarized, and included in the NDA, which is submitted to FDA. If, after review, FDA approves the NDA, the pharmaceutical company may choose to market the drug. Even after marketing begins, however, additional information on the safety and efficacy of the drug will be gathered as physicians, the pharmaceutical industry, and FDA continue to monitor for toxicity, side effects, further benefits, and other indications. Data obtained are shared among health professionals through mailings or publications, and indeed may cause the modification of product data and use where deemed essential.

The formal postmarketing study of a drug may also take place in what is known as a Phase IV study. Phase IV studies are not mandated in FDA regulations but are discussed in FDA guidelines. A Phase IV study may be a condition of FDA approval to market a drug if the uncertainty about a drug's safety or efficacy does not warrant delaying its release on the market, or it may be initiated by a pharmaceutical company to further substantiate drug safety and efficacy and to support marketing claims (IOM, 1985). Phase IV studies may be controlled or observational.

## REFERENCES

EPA (U.S. Environmental Protection Agency). 1984. Guidelines Subdivision F—Hazard Evaluation: Human and Domestic Animals, revised ed. Washington, D.C.: EPA.

IOM (Institute of Medicine). 1985. Assessing Medical Technologies. Washington, D.C.: National Academy Press.

Wierenga, D.E., and Eaton, C.R. 1993. The drug development and approval process. In: In Development: New Medicines for Older Americans. Washington, D.C.: Pharmaceutical Manufacturers Association.

# 2

# Women's Participation in Clinical Studies

In recent years, both scientific and public attention has focused on the level of women's participation in clinical studies and on the position of women's health issues in the national research agenda. In a spate of articles in professional journals, authors have criticized "gaps in medical knowledge" about women, questioned how the "white male [came] to be the prototype of the human research subject," and commented on "gender disparit[ies] in our scientific and medical knowledge base" (Cotton, 1990b; Dresser, 1992; Sherman, 1993; see also Cotton, 1990a, 1992; Healy, 1991; Gurwitz et al., 1992; Johnson, 1992). Coverage in newspapers and popular magazines, including the *New York Times, Washington Post,* and *Washingtonian,* has added to the level of interest in these issues (Kolata, 1990; Okie, 1990; Herman, 1992; Stevens, 1992; McGuire, 1993).

The current concern about women's participation in clinical studies arises from the conflict of two public policy positions: the need to protect research participants and the "rights" of participants to access clinical studies. The roots of protectionism go deeper than those of greater access. For example, in the wake of revelations that government-funded research projects engaged in unethical treatment of participants (see below), policies were formulated to protect human volunteers. Policies grounded in protectionist considerations contributed to the later exclusion of pregnant women and women of childbearing potential from some clinical studies, most notably, early-phase drug trials. Protectionist policies do not adequately account, however, for what many perceive to be the relative inattention to the study of health problems experienced primarily by women. This alleged inattention may arise from subtler (yet powerful) forces such as gender and race biases that permeate both society and scientific research (see Chapter 5).

Contributing to the current focus on access to health care and health research are a wide range of factors, including the emergence of human rights movements to represent the concerns of diverse racial and ethnic groups, women, gays, lesbians, and persons with disabilities; the growing funding of biomedical research; the advent of new medical technologies to diagnose, prevent, and cure disease; and the public availability of information about these medical advances. In particular, the spread of acquired immune deficiency syndrome (AIDS) and the activism of health advocacy groups representing diverse populations have served to focus attention on the extent of scientific knowledge and research concerning the health problems of women and racial and ethnic groups.

## HISTORICAL BACKGROUND

As part of its study of federal policies, the committee traced the evolution of the current standards governing the participation of women (and men) in clinical studies. The history begins with the early attempts to deal with ethical aspects of the use of human research participants. These efforts led to a period of public policy dominated by a protectionist agenda that is now being replaced by an emerging emphasis on expanded access to clinical studies. The present, rapidly changing policy environment is a product of professional and governmental policy responses to: (1) identified abuses in the use of human participants; (2) more recent changes in the public policy dialogue and in drug development and the corresponding governmental policy responses, primarily by the Food and Drug Administration (FDA); and (3) the role of both women's health and AIDS advocates in drawing attention to what they perceived to be inequitable research practices and the relative absence of women and racial and ethnic groups from the research agenda. This historical context gave the committee a better understanding of the rationale behind its charge, and therefore a better understanding of some the subtleties of the legal and ethical issues.

### Evolution of Protectionist Policies

Policy development in the area of protection of human research subjects began in 1949 with the issuance of the Nuremberg Code, which outlined standards for the judgment of flagrantly abusive human experimentation conducted by the Nazis in World War II. The code articulated ten basic principles regarding moral, ethical, and legal requirements of research involving human subjects, including the provisions that research subjects must have the legal capacity to give consent, the ability to exercise free power of choice, and sufficient knowledge and comprehension to be able to make an informed decision. The code also dictated that experiments involving human subjects should yield useful results that cannot be achieved by other methods, avoid unnecessary suffering and injury, assure that risk does not exceed importance, and be done by scientifically qualified persons with adequate facilities for subject protection. Further, the code stipulated that human subjects be at liberty to withdraw from the study at any time and that the scientist be prepared to terminate the experiment if continuation is likely to result in injury, disability, or death to the subject.

The Nuremberg Code provided a model for later statements regarding research on human subjects, including the Declaration of Helsinki Recommendations Guiding Medical Doctors in Biomedical Research Involving Human Subjects, first adopted in 1964. A more immediate reaction to the Nuremberg Code, however, was evident in the formulation of guidelines for clinical research at the Clinical Center of the NIH, a research hospital opened in 1953. Titled "Group Considerations for Clinical Research Procedures Deviating from Accepted Medical Practice or Involving Universal Hazards," these guidelines were the first federal guidelines for human studies research and the first official statement requiring committee review of human studies protocols.

## Research Abuses

In the 1960s and 1970s, several unfortunate events demonstrated that serious problems remained with regard to the protection of human research subjects. Landmark research abuses, including those involving elderly, debilitated patients and African Americans, signaled the desperate need for the clarification and, more important, the formalization of existing guidelines for human subjects research. While the Nuremberg Code and Declaration of Helsinki were well known, they included no explicit provisions for enforcement.

The vulnerability of the elderly to research abuse was highlighted in 1963, when it was discovered that a physician at the Jewish Chronic Disease Hospital in Brooklyn, New York, was experimentally injecting live cancer cells into elderly debilitated patients without proper informed consent. Review proceedings indicated that the study, designed to explore the immune system's role in defense against cancer, had not been presented to the hospital's research committee and that several physicians responsible for the subjects' care had not been consulted before the injections were given (Faden and Beauchamp, 1986). It was also revealed that the physicians who *had* been consulted prior to the experiment had argued against the research on the basis that the patients were incapable of giving informed consent.

The failure to properly obtain consent at the Jewish Chronic Disease Hospital was not an isolated case. In 1965 Henry K. Beecher, a Harvard anesthesiologist, gave a highly publicized speech that highlighted cases in the published literature of neglect of the consent process in human subjects research. In this speech, and in a subsequent paper, he recounted several examples of studies in which subjects had not received satisfactory explanations of risks. Beecher stated, "it must be apparent that they would not have been available if they had been truly aware of the uses that would be made of them" (Beecher, 1966). Although Beecher realized that he risked criticism for exposing these abuses, he believed strongly that such abuses not only had grave consequences for the subjects, but for the medical profession as well.

In February of the following year, Surgeon General William H. Stewart responded to these revelations by requiring that all extramural research supported by the U.S. Public Health Service be subject to review by an independent committee of institutional associates. These committees were to include members of the community as well as scientists, and they would assure that the proposed informed consent procedures were adequate. These requirements did not, however, have the force of regulations.

In the early 1970s, the abuses of the infamous Tuskegee Syphilis Study were revealed, adding fuel to arguments that human research subjects were not being adequately protected by the existing guidelines, and that more formal *regulations* were in order. This observational study of untreated syphilis, begun in 1932, involved approximately 400 African American men, many of whom were allowed to remain untreated for the disease, even after antibiotic treatment was widely available (Jones, 1981; King, 1992). There was no evidence that informed consent was received from the subjects. Because the study was initiated before the Nuremberg Code, it had not been subject to any "ethical" review; funding for the study had simply been renewed over the years in accordance with the recommendations of the investigators.

Shortly after these abuses were revealed, a congressional panel was convened to review the study's history and to recommend appropriate action by the federal government. In its final report the panel concluded that the study had been ethically unjustifiable from its inception, that it should be immediately disbanded, and that all surviving study subjects should be located and treated (USDHEW, 1973). The panel also expressed concern that "no uniform departmental policy for the protection of research subjects exist[ed]" for government-sponsored research. Finally, the panel recommended that the Department of Health, Education, and Welfare (DHEW) standards regarding informed consent of research subjects be clarified and that an effective enforcement mechanism be devised.

On May 30, 1974, existing guidelines for the protection of human research subjects finally took the shape of federal regulations. Promulgated by DHEW, the regulations established the institutional review board (IRB), a more formal version of the research review committee, as one mechanism for the protection of human research subjects. The responsibilities given to IRBs included the reviewing of risk-benefit ratios, confidentiality protections, informed consent processes and documents, and procedures for selection of subjects (to ensure that selection is equitable).

## Responses to Fetal Injury

In the 1960s and 1970s, as the country was coping with the events at the Jewish Chronic Disease Hospital and Tuskegee, problems caused by two medications, thalidomide and diethylstilbestrol (DES), would amplify public sentiment about the need for greater protection for fetuses from risks in science and medicine. These concerns were ultimately translated into protective policies directed toward women of childbearing potential, including pregnant women.

Thalidomide, approved for marketing in 1958, was used primarily as a sedative and antidote for nausea in early pregnancy. The drug was approved for over-the-counter sale in 20 countries (not including the United States) and was widely used. While marketing approval had been delayed in this country, many U.S. women received thalidomide from "investigating" doctors who had been given the drug by the manufacturer. As thalidomide was being widely distributed, physicians began to note a startling increase in the number of children born with a rare set of deformities, the most prominent features of which were severe limb malformations (Christie, 1962). By 1962, when sufficient statistical evidence had accumulated to establish thalidomide as the causative agent of these deformities, approximately 8,000 children had been affected.

The blame for what is often referred to as the "thalidomide disaster" is alleged to reside in inadequate research standards, a failure of the drug's manufacturer to acknowledge early evidence of side effects and reports that were critical of the drug, and physicians' uncritical acceptance of promotional claims (Levine, 1993). The response from the U.S. science establishment was the creation of new legislation: the Kefauver-Harris amendments of 1962. These amendments to the drug approval laws instituted a rigorous preapproval process at the FDA. Although the "thalidomide disaster" did not result from women's participation in research, the experience had a powerful emotional impact that created an aversion to involving pregnant women and women of childbearing age in drug research (Levine, 1993). The DES experience would bolster this aversion.

DES is a synthetic hormone that was widely prescribed in the 1940s and 1950s to prevent miscarriage (see DES Case Study in Appendix C). Enthusiastic physicians overlooked large, controlled clinical trials indicating that DES was ineffective. They focused instead on smaller studies in which the drug appeared to show promise (Levine, 1993). It was not until 20 years later, in the late 1960s and early 1970s, that the side effects of the drug would become evident: the daughters of women who had taken DES during pregnancy began to experience a rare adenocarcinoma of the vagina. Public trust in science and medicine was shaken once again, and a protectionist stance toward including fertile women in drug trials became further entrenched. Although the DES claims were based on injuries incurred in the context of medical practice, not in the context of formal research, the substantial costs incurred by pharmaceutical companies through DES-related litigation encouraged the practice of excluding pregnant and potentially pregnant women from clinical research. FDA guidelines issued in the late 1970s would serve to reinforce this exclusionary practice.

In July of 1974, Congress passed the National Research Act (P.L. 93-348), which called for the establishment of a National Commission for the Protection of Human Subjects of Biomedical and Behavioral Research (National Commission) to "identify ethical principles" and to "develop guidelines" for research involving human subjects. This commission operated between 1974 and 1978 and issued many reports. In 1975, guidelines developed by the National Commission for research on fetuses and pregnant women were incorporated into DHHS regulations for research on human subjects. These federal regulations, still in effect today, identify the limited conditions under which an IRB may approve research on pregnant women and fetuses (see Chapter 6). Subsequent regulations instituted to protect children and prisoners from research abuses have served to group pregnant women in the category of "vulnerable populations," a designation that is reinforced by current regulatory language (see 45 C.F.R. 46.111[a][3]). This grouping has been criticized for its implication that pregnant women are incapable of making responsible decisions for themselves and future offspring.

Although DHHS included restrictions on the inclusion of women of childbearing potential in earlier drafts of the regulation concerning pregnant women, these references were eliminated from the final regulation. In 1977, however, FDA issued guidelines for drug development that recommended that women of childbearing potential be excluded from early phases of drug trials (except in the case of life-threatening diseases).

## Advent of Inclusionary Policies

The publication of the National Commission's *Belmont Report* in 1978 was a watershed event in the shift away from practices and policies that some might label "paternalistic" toward greater valuation of the autonomy of research subjects. The *Belmont Report* identified three comprehensive ethical principles that provide an analytical framework for scientists, physicians, research subjects, and reviewers of research proposals to understand the ethical issues inherent in humans subjects research. The three principles were: (1) respect for persons (individuals should be treated as autonomous agents and persons with diminished autonomy are entitled to protection); (2) beneficence (maximize possible benefits and minimize possible harms); and (3) justice (fairness in the selection of subjects for clinical research) (National Commission, 1978). Events of the following decade would sharpen this focus on the rights of research subjects.

In the 1980s, AIDS activists working to promote access to experimental AIDS therapies offered the first formal challenge to the protectionist policies of the preceding decades (Rothman and Edgar, 1992). Frustrated with the length of time required for new drugs to move through the FDA approval process, these activists called for a new mechanism for earlier release of AIDS drugs in the development process (Levi, 1991). In May of 1987, the FDA issued regulations that expanded access to experimental drugs used to treat serious and life-threatening illnesses (Rothman and Edgar, 1990). As described below, the success of AIDS activists would serve to energize the women's health movement.

At roughly the same time the AIDS "movement" was born, advocates for women's health began to call for more focused research on health problems unique to women. Women had united around health concerns in the 1970s, a movement exemplified by the publication of *Our Bodies, Ourselves* (Boston Women's Health Book Collective, 1973), a women's health care manual created in reaction to a health care system that many women perceived to be unresponsive to their needs. In the 1980s, however, women gained sufficient political power to forcefully confront the science and health bureaucracy.

In the late 1980s, women of the baby boom generation began to reach mid-life and to experience menopause and breast and reproductive cancers. The perception of a relative lack of attention to women's health in the scientific and medical establishment became of increasingly salient concern to this group of women. Better educated and employed in more powerful positions than their predecessors, baby boom women began to take action by supporting female political candidates, fund-raising for women's issues, and forming interest groups to educate themselves and to pressure unresponsive bureaucrats—the very strategies AIDS activists had used with success. In addition, dramatic increases in medical school enrollment among women during the 1970s (AMA, 1991) began to produce a vocal group of medical professionals who questioned current priorities and policies in women's health research.

Many observers have pointed to the 1985 report of the U.S. Public Health Service Task Force on Women's Health Issues as the cornerstone of the current focus on biomedical research in the women's health movement (Auerbach, 1993; Johnson, 1994). This task force concluded that:

> The historical lack of research focus on women's health concerns has compromised the quality of health information available to women as well as the health care they receive [U.S. Public Health Service, 1985].

The accompanying recommendations ultimately provoked NIH to announce a new policy in 1986 that urged funding applicants to include women in clinical research. The policy also stated that applicants should provide a clear rationale for proposed exclusions of women and that investigators should evaluate gender differences in their findings. The Alcohol, Drug Abuse, and Mental Health Administration, another agency of the U.S. Public Health Service, co-sponsored the policy (GAO, 1990).

Public attention to the issue of women's inclusion in clinical research and the implications of this inclusion for the status of women's health gained tremendous momentum in 1990 when the General Accounting Office (GAO) released a report in which it evaluated the efficacy of the 1986 NIH policy. In congressional testimony regarding this report, a GAO representative stated that the unautomated, decentralized recordkeeping at NIH had prevented GAO from systematically evaluating the effectiveness of the NIH policy. He concluded that "NIH [had] no way to measure the policy's impact on the research it funds" (GAO, 1990). GAO also reported that the 1986 policy had not been well disseminated internally to individual institutes or centers, nor to prospective grant applicants, and therefore probably had not been implemented consistently, if at all. In addition, the GAO pointed to some of the larger, more expensive NIH-funded clinical studies that had included only men as evidence of the ineffectiveness of the policy. One of the examples was the Physician's Health Study, an all-male study of the role of aspirin in the prevention of heart attacks.

## NIH Office of Research on Women's Health and Recent Changes

Following the release of the 1990 GAO report, women's health advocacy groups and other organizations initiated their own efforts to clarify the picture of women's participation in clinical research (AMA Council on Ethical and Judicial Affairs, 1991; IOM, 1991a; PMA, 1991). A significant shift in popular opinion, however, already had begun to develop. Practices and policies once presented as protective were now labeled as paternalistic and discriminatory. The rationales behind a number of clinical studies that had proceeded without question were now being challenged. Why had the NIH-sponsored Multiple Risk-Factor Intervention Trials (MRFIT) of heart disease not included women when women as well as men were dying of heart disease? How could the Baltimore Longitudinal Study of Aging include no women when the elderly population in this country is disproportionately female?

In September 1990, largely in response to the impact of the GAO report, Acting NIH Director William Raub announced the creation of the NIH Office of Research on Women's Health (ORWH). Located within the director's office, ORWH was given a three-part mandate:

> 1. to strengthen and enhance research related to diseases, disorders, and conditions that affect women and to ensure that research conducted and supported by NIH adequately addresses issues regarding women's health;
>
> 2. to ensure that women are appropriately represented in biomedical and behavioral research studies supported by NIH; and
>
> 3. to foster the increased enrollment of women in biomedical research—especially in pivotal decisionmaking roles within both clinical medicine and the research environment [NIH, 1992b].

Although the ORWH began its work almost immediately, it would not be statutorily authorized until June 1993.

The legislation that would eventually authorize the ORWH as a permanent entity began as part of the Women's Health Equity Act (WHEA), an omnibus legislative package first introduced in July 1990 by Representatives Schroeder and Snowe. Reintroduced in 1991, the WHEA contained 22 bills that addressed research, care, and prevention issues in women's health. During the 1991–1992 legislative year, six of the research-related provisions of the WHEA (including the provision to permanently authorize the ORWH) were incorporated into the NIH Revitalization Act, which reauthorizes the programs of the NIH. These provisions authorized additional funding for breast cancer, ovarian and other reproductive cancers, and osteoporosis and related bone disorders; they also called for the establishment of three contraceptive research centers and two fertility research centers. One of the provisions included a policy regarding inclusion of women and racial and ethnic groups in NIH-sponsored or -funded clinical research.

The NIH Revitalization Act passed both the Senate and the House of Representatives, only to be vetoed by President Bush in June 1992 because of provisions that called for lifting of the moratorium on federally funded fetal tissue transplantation research. With strong support from Senate Majority Leader George Mitchell, the bill was introduced, with the women's health provisions intact, in January 1993. President Clinton, who had vowed during his presidential campaign to overturn the fetal tissue transplantation moratorium, signed the NIH Revitalization Act into law on June 10, 1993.

In 1991 both NIH and the Alcohol, Drug Abuse, and Mental Health Administration (ADAMHA)[1] issued special instructions to grant applicants directing that women and racial and ethnic groups be included in clinical study populations. The instructions also stated that clear and compelling rationales for the exclusion of women and racial and ethnic groups should accompany proposals that do not include these groups. NIH also devised a plan to facilitate the implementation of the new policy; it included educational programs for reviewers, investigators, and NIH staff and for a coding system to track gender and racial and ethnic group representation in extramural clinical studies. (See Chapter 6.)

Later in 1991, Bernadine Healy, the first woman director of NIH, announced NIH's plans to initiate a major longitudinal study of women's health, called the Women's Health Initiative (WHI). A 14-year, $625 million research initiative, the WHI would address the preventive effects of smoking cessation, exercise, hormone therapy, diet, and dietary supplements on osteoporosis, cancer, and cardiovascular disease in postmenopausal women.

In addition to the policy changes at NIH, events outside the federal science and health establishment stirred public sentiment about paternalism, protectionism, and discrimination. In 1991, the U.S. Supreme Court heard *International Union, UAW v. Johnson Controls,* a case involving a battery manufacturing company (Johnson Controls, Inc.) that had a policy barring women of reproductive age from performing certain jobs because of the potential risk of fetal injury and subsequent company liability. The Court ruled that this policy constituted sex discrimination and was therefore unconstitutional (see Chapter 6). Many policy analysts would add that the sexual harassment hearings that preceded Clarence Thomas' confirmation to the Supreme Court also heightened sensitivity to issues of gender in politics (Auerbach, 1993).

Since the initiation of this committee's deliberations in the fall of 1992, a number of additional events have taken place that have influenced women's inclusion in clinical studies. In October 1992, FDA cosponsored a conference with the Food and Drug Law Institute (FDLI) on issues related to the inclusion of women in clinical trials of FDA-related products (Women in Clinical Trials of FDA-Regulated Products, Washington, D.C., 5 October). A primary purpose of the conference was to discuss the FDA's 1977 guidelines, particularly as they pertained to exclusion of "women of childbearing potential" from early phases of most new drug trials.

Later in October of 1992, the GAO released a second report that addressed the inclusion of women in clinical studies. The report examined the FDA's policies and the pharmaceutical industry's practices regarding experimental drug testing in women. The report's conclusions were based on the results of a questionnaire sent by the GAO to each pharmaceutical company that had secured FDA approval for a new drug between January 1988 and June 1991. The questionnaire requested information about the extent of women's inclusion in new drug studies and efforts to detect and analyze gender differences (GAO, 1992).

The GAO states in the report that although women were included in most of the drug studies reported, "for more than 60 percent of the drugs, the representation of women in the test population was less than the representation of women in the population with the corresponding disease" (GAO, 1992). Representation of women was found to be particularly poor in cardiovascular drug trials, a finding the GAO noted "with particular concern" because this is an area in which gender differences in drug response had been observed. In addition, the GAO indicated that pharmaceutical manufacturers frequently failed to analyze trial data for gender differences, despite an FDA guideline that encourages gender analysis. Although FDA and industry representatives have expressed some agreement with GAO's findings, particularly with respect to the conduct of gender analyses, many have disputed GAO's definition of "representative" numbers of women (FDA, 1992).

On March 24, 1993, the FDA announced the lifting of the 1977 restriction on the inclusion of women of childbearing potential in early clinical trials, including pharmacology studies and early therapeutic studies. Issued officially in the *Federal Register* on July 22, 1993, the revised FDA policy also formalized its expectations regarding analysis of clinical data by gender, assessment of potential pharmacokinetic differences between genders, and, where appropriate, assessment of pharmacodynamic differences and the conduct of specific additional studies in women (FDA, 1993b). A major intent of the new guideline is to give more flexibility to IRBs, investigators, and subjects in determining how best to ensure the safe and scientifically valid participation of women of reproductive potential in clinical studies.

NIH has also been active. In March 1993, ORWH sponsored a public hearing on recruitment and retention of women in clinical studies. A task force on recruitment and retention of women in clinical studies has worked throughout the year to develop recommendations to NIH. Another relevant NIH report currently under way is an official progress report on the inclusion of women and racial and ethnic groups in NIH-sponsored research, a report prepared as a follow-up to the 1990 GAO report. This report will include an analysis of data collected from all NIH institutes since the institution of the 1991 policy regarding the inclusion of women and racial and ethnic groups in clinical studies.

Recently NIH announced plans to convene a conference to discuss the establishment of a database for tracking and monitoring clinical trials data, including data on gender composition. These efforts are a response to a provision of the NIH Revitalization Act that requires NIH to establish a national data system and clearinghouse for research on women's health. The provision states that the data system must include a "registry of clinical trials of experimental treatments that have been developed for women's health" and that the registry must include information on "subject eligibility criteria, sex, age, ethnicity or race, and the location of trial site or sites." Finally, it mandates timely reporting of new trials and trial results by investigators.

These recent activities are evidence of the growing realization in the scientific and political communities that policies designed to protect certain populations from research risk may actually expose these populations to a greater risk of another kind: a lack of data about their health. There has been a forceful movement in recent years away from these protectionist policies: Chapter 6 describes current federal policies that encourage— and sometimes require—the inclusion of previously unrepresented or underrepresented groups. Similarly, Chapters 3, 4, and 5 summarize the social, ethical, and scientific arguments that have helped to form this emerging consensus. All of these arguments return us to a very important question: Are women currently underrepresented in federally sponsored clinical research?

## CURRENT STATUS

Attempts to determine whether women have participated in the whole of clinical studies to the same extent as men, and whether women have been disadvantaged by policies and practices regarding their participation or by a failure to focus on their health interests in the conduct of research, are hindered by a scarcity of reported data. Despite the growing literature on women and biomedical research, no truly comprehensive analysis of these issues has been published. This sort of analysis would be easier to accomplish if a centralized database of clinical study information (including both the research questions addressed and the gender composition of subject populations) was in place. Unfortunately, as discussed in a later section, there is no such centralized registry of clinical studies conducted in the United States. Several specialized registries are in operation, but they are not easily accessible to researchers or to the general public. And, in the case of at least one clinical study registry, information on gender composition of study populations was not collected until relatively recently.

When GAO sought to ascertain the extent of NIH implementation of its 1986 policy on the inclusion of women in clinical studies, it found that NIH did not maintain consistent records on participation by gender. Nevertheless, based on examination of some of the larger NIH-sponsored studies, GAO concluded in its 1990 report that NIH had not fully implemented the policy, and that indeed women were "generally underrepresented" in the drug trials it examined. GAO again encountered data collection problems in researching its 1992 report on FDA policies and the pharmaceutical industry's practices regarding research on women in prescription drug testing. Because FDA did not maintain easily accessible records on gender composition of study populations, GAO chose to survey pharmaceutical companies directly. GAO concluded that women were "generally underrepresented" in the drug trials it examined and that trial data were not adequately analyzed for gender differences. It is important to note here that FDA and PMA do not necessarily accept GAO's definition of the term "underrepresentation," and thus disagree that women have been underrepresented in such trials.

The committee did not have the resources even to begin to address the "bottom line" question of whether the health of women has been less well served by the biomedical research community than the health of men. The committee did attempt, however, to determine the extent of women's overall participation in clinical studies through a survey of the published scientific literature. The committee identified a number of papers that address the issue of the participation of women as subjects in clinical or social science research (see Appendix A of this volume). These papers include published and unpublished literature reviews, reviews of current protocols across institutions, surveys of research at individual institutions, surveys of research conducted by pharmaceutical companies, and testimony from agency officials. Some of the papers focus on research targeted at specific conditions such as heart disease or AIDS; others consider the broader spectrum of human subjects research in the social sciences as well as in medicine.

The committee also initiated several analyses of available information on clinical study subject populations. One committee member who serves as chair of an IRB collected information on the gender composition of subject populations in studies approved by all of his institution's IRBs within the last two years. The committee also analyzed data from an NIH clinical study inventory that operated for a short time in the late 1970s. In addition, the committee commissioned retrospective surveys of clinical studies reported in two scientific journals, the *Journal of the American Medical Association* (Bird, 1994) and *Controlled Clinical Trials* (Meinert, 1993a). These studies are summarized in Table 2-1 and described in Appendix A to this volume.

The sources of information available to the committee vary widely in scope and method, which makes the data difficult to synthesize. All of the sources provide some kind of data on women's participation in clinical studies, but many do not provide the kinds of information that would allow the committee to make a judgment about the appropriateness of the reported study composition (e.g., condition under study, percentages of male and female subjects included in studies of conditions affecting both males and females, adequacy of sample size to analyze gender differences). In addition, much of this evidence could be colored by the publishing preferences of both authors and editors.

As can be seen from Table 2-1, the available evidence is insufficient to determine whether women have participated in the whole of clinical studies to the same extent as men, and whether women have been disadvantaged by policies and practices regarding their participation or a failure to focus on their health interest in the conduct of research (see Appendix A for complete descriptions of studies). Some studies found that an appropriate number of women were included in specific study populations and that more female-only studies were being conducted than male-only studies. Others found that women were "over-" or "underrepresented" in certain types of studies. Others found that women—especially elderly or poor women of diverse racial and ethnic groups—are less likely to be included in studies than men. The committee can conclude from this survey that there are many unanswered questions about gender-based differences in response to treatment, and that investigators may not have done one or more of the following: reported the results of gender analyses, performed gender analyses of study results, or recruited adequate numbers of women to support the kind of subgroup analysis that would be needed to resolve these questions. During the preparation of this report, the committee was advised that ORWH was preparing a follow-up report to the 1990 GAO report that summarizes clinical study data collected since 1991, when the NIH implemented an improved coding system for tracking and reporting data on gender and racial and ethnic group representation in all NIH-funded clinical studies. The ORWH report was not yet available when this report went to press.

Even the best database, it should be emphasized, is incapable in and of itself of supplying answers to the question of whether women are being treated fairly, compared to men, by the research enterprise. Such a judgment is necessarily based on complex, value-based criteria that influence interpretation of the data. Data about participation by gender may not reveal whether any particular gender-based interests in a study or field of research are being served, or how well.

## Studies of Heart Disease and AIDS

Although the committee was unable to establish that gender inequity existed in the whole of past clinical research, it was able to find evidence relevant to this issue in two areas of disease research: AIDS and heart disease. In both fields, there is some evidence of studies that either exclude women altogether or include them in numbers too small to yield meaningful information about their treatment—although there is not necessarily agreement that these practices were either scientifically or ethically inappropri-

TABLE 2-1 Findings and Conclusions of Previous Studies of Women's Participation in Clinical Studies

| Reference | Source | Type | Coverage | Findings and Author's Conclusions |
|---|---|---|---|---|
| Reardon and Prescott, 1977 | Journal | Literature review | One 1972 volume and one 1974 volume of the *Journal of Personality and Social Psychology* | Decrease in percentage of all-male studies; increase in the percentage of all-female studies; increase in gender analysis for both-sex studies |
| Prescott, 1978 | Journal | Literature review and interview survey | *Journal of Personality and Social Psychology*, 1970 and 1971 | The author interviewed 62 researchers who had authored 64 single-sex studies. Replies were analyzed for thematic content and formed three major types: "scientific" (e.g., "desire to reduce the variation in subject' responses"; 56 percent), "practical" (e.g., "limited money and resources for dealing with an increased sample size"; 28 percent), and "extra-scientific" (e.g., "lack of interest in questions related to sex differences"; 15 percent). There has been an imbalance in psychology that has led to the study of men rather than women or both sexes. |
| Kinney et al., 1981 | Journal | Literature review | 50 Clinical trials reported in 1979 | Young women served less frequently than young men as subjects in premarketing clinical drug trials. Women are underrepresented in new drug trials. |
| GAO, 1990 | Government publication | Data review | 50 Current NIH grant applications | Twenty percent of proposals provided no information about the gender of study participants; over one-third of proposals indicated that both genders would be included, but did not specify proportions; several proposals for all-male studies provided no rationale for single-sex design. NIH had not successfully |

| | | | | implemented its 1986 policy encouraging: (1) inclusion of women in study populations and (2) justification for studies proposing to exclude women. |
|---|---|---|---|---|
| Hooper, 1990 | Government publication | Data review | Women enrolled in 5 categories of randomized-control trial | Women appear to be included in trials of AIDS drugs in a proportion that approximates the proportion of people with AIDS who are women. Women appear to be slightly "overrepresented" in trials of nicotine gum for smoking cessation. Women appear to be "underrepresented" in clinical studies of antiplatelet drugs for preventing stroke, anti-hypertensives, and drugs for myocardial infarction. |
| NIH, National Heart, Lung, and Blood Institute (NHLBI), 1990 | Government publication | Data review | NHLBI-initiated epidemiologic and primary prevention trials active in 1990 | Found 2 trials included exclusively women; 3 included between 30 and 45 percent women; 10 included between 50 and 58 percent women; and 3 included exclusively men. |
| Cotton, 1990b | Journal | Literature review | Multiple Risk Factor Intervention Trials (MRFIT); Physicians Health Study; "all the large trials of cholesterol-lowering drugs" that include only men | There are important gaps in knowledge about the medical treatment of women, the elderly, and nonwhite persons despite mounting documentation of differences in drug responses and risk profiles among these cohorts. |
| Edwards, 1991 | Pharmaceutical industry publication | Questionnaire | Questionnaire sent to 46 of the largest pharmaceutical companies (33 responses) | All 33 companies reported that they collect data on gender of trial participants (94 percent always; 6 percent usually); 25 of the 33 companies reported that they deliberately recruit "representative" numbers of women for clinical trials. |

(*continued*)

TABLE 2-1 Continued

| Reference | Source | Type | Coverage | Findings and Author's Conclusions |
|---|---|---|---|---|
| Ungerleider and Friedman, 1991 | Government publication | Data review | 444 Treatment protocols active in January 1991 within the National Cancer Institute's Clinical Trials Cooperative Group Program | The only protocols that specified gender of subjects were those for drugs to treat sex-specific cancers (with the exception of breast cancer protocols, which excluded men). |
| IOM, 1991a | Unpublished conference summary | Data review | 907 Grants (ADAMHA) | Found 12 percent of grants represented research including only women; 18 percent included only men; 70 percent included women and men; when all grants were considered together, women comprised 53 percent of the total study population. |
| PMA, 1991 | Pharmaceutical industry publication | Data review | Medicines in development as of December 1991 (no total given) | Noted 263 drugs were under development for use in women (to treat diseases that affect only women, that disproportionately affect women, or are one of the top 10 causes of death in women). The top three areas of drug development were cancer (58 medicines), gynecologic diseases (51 medicines), and cardiovascular/cerebrovascular disease (48 medicines). "America's pharmaceutical research companies recognize the unique medical needs of women and . . . are working hard to resolve the difficulties of developing drugs to meet those needs." |
| Levey, 1991 | Journal | Literature review | Clinical trials reported in all January issues of *Clinical Pharmacology & Therapeutics* (CP&T) between 1981 and 1991 | The author compared trials reported in the 1981 and 1991 January issues of CP&T and found a decline in the number of trials restricted to male subjects and a more than twofold increase in the number of |

| | | | | trials that included both men and women. When the author extended the survey to trials reported in all January issues of *CP&T* between 1981 and 1991, no consistent pattern (i.e., increase or decrease) emerged for studies that included both men and women. Further investigation is required to conclude definitely that there has been a true progression toward an appropriate balance of men and women as research participants in studies published in *CP&T* in the past decade. |
|---|---|---|---|---|
| Dresser, 1992 | Journal | Literature review | Select large-scale NIH-sponsored studies | The failure to include women in clinical research populations is ubiquitous. |
| Larson, In press | Journal | Data review | Research protocols approved by an IRB at a major tertiary care center during 1989 and 1990 | Women were not "underrepresented" in clinical drug trials or other types of research. Age, race, and socioeconomic status were more likely than gender to be associated with an unjustified exclusion from research protocols. |
| Gannon et al., 1992 | Journal | Literature review | 4,952 Articles published in sample years between 1970 and 1990 in the areas of developmental, physiological, and social psychology | Significant increases in the number of female first authors and participants; significant decreases in sexist language and inappropriate generalization from males to females. Despite improvements, data reveal continued evidence of discriminatory practices. |

*(continued)*

TABLE 2-1 Continued

| Reference | Source | Type | Coverage | Findings and Author's Conclusions |
|---|---|---|---|---|
| Gurwitz et al., 1992 | Journal | Literature review | All studies of specific pharmacotherapies employed in the treatment of acute myocardial infarction that appeared in the English-language literature between January 1960 and September 1991 | Age-based exclusions are frequently used in clinical trials of these pharmacotherapies. Age-based exclusions limit the ability to generalize study findings to the patient population that experiences the most morbidity and mortality from acute myocardial infarction: persons over age 75. Because women outlive men by an average of 7.5 years, they are disproportionately represented in the elderly population. |
| PMA, 1992a | Pharmaceutical industry publication | Data review | 91 Clinical trials active in October 1992 of medicines for AIDS and AIDS-related conditions | Of the 91 medicines, 50 included women in human clinical trials and 13 medicines included children in trials. |
| GAO, 1992 | Government publication | Data review | All drug manufacturers that obtained FDA approval between January 1988 and June 1991 for drugs combining new chemical properties | One-quarter of drug manufacturers did not deliberately recruit "representative" number of women as participants in drug trials; for more then 60 percent of the drugs in the survey, the representation of women was less than in the population with the corresponding disease; for about one-third of the drugs, fewer than 250 women (the minimum number suggested by FDA) were included as participants. Women were included in trials for all the drugs in the survey but were generally "underrepresented" in the trials. Most trials did not include enough women to permit the detection of gender-related differences in drug |

| | | | | response. Even when there were enough women included in trials, trial data were seldom analyzed for gender differences in response. In addition, many drug manufacturers did not study whether their drugs interact with hormones present in women, including hormonal contraceptives. |
|---|---|---|---|---|
| PMA, 1992b | Pharmaceutical industry publication | Data review | Orphan drugs under development in October 1992 | 26 Orphan products were in development for diseases that exclusively or predominantly affect women; for all trials of orphan drugs, enrollment of women approximates the prevalence in women of the disease under study. Women are adequately represented in trials of orphan drugs. |
| Williams and Manace Borins, 1993 | Journal | Literature review | 160 Randomly selected articles from the 1989 *New England Journal of Medicine* | 16 Components of the research process were examined for gender bias: significant (present in greater than 60 percent of the articles) gender bias was found for 12 of the 16 components examined. Medical research in 1989 was seriously gender-biased, and therefore scientifically flawed. |
| Pham et al., 1992 | Interest group publication | Data review | AIDS Clinical Trial Group (ACTG) clinical trials | Women, intravenous drug users, people of color, and people of low income have been grossly underrepresented among study subjects in ACTG clinical trials. |
| Charo, 1992 | Unpublished paper | Data review | All drug study protocols submitted for review to the Human Subject Committee of the University of Wisconsin in 1989 and 1990 | Of 169 studies, 28 (16.5 percent) excluded fertile women; 22 of these 28 studies were sponsored by pharmaceutical companies. |

(continued)

TABLE 2-1 Continued

| Reference | Source | Type | Coverage | Findings and Author's Conclusions |
|---|---|---|---|---|
| NOW Legal Defense and Education Fund, 1993 | Interest group statement | Data review | ACTG clinical trials, 1990-1992 | The percentage of female enrollment in these trials increased from 6.5 percent to 7.8 percent between 1990 and 1992; of 74 AIDS clinical trials open for enrollment in New York and New Jersey in October 1990, 57 (80 percent) specifically excluded pregnant women. The numbers of women enrolled in ACTG trials are not great enough to provide sound and meaningful data on the effects of a given drug in women. Pregnant women are under-represented in trials of AIDS drugs. |
| Long, 1993 | Testimony prepared for government hearing | Data review | ACTG clinical trials, as of January 1993 | The percentage of women accrued as ACTG trial participants (10.3) is slightly less than women's percentage (10.9) of CDC-reported AIDS cases; only two trials restricted enrollment exclusively to women, and both focused on prevention of transmission of HIV to the fetus; percentages of women were as low as 5.3 percent in important opportunistic infection therapy trials. Women seem to be represented in ACTG clinical trials in proportion to the incidence of AIDS among women. Women have been underrepresented in trials of drugs for AIDS-related opportunistic infections. |
| Eichler et al., 1992 | Journal | Literature review | Selected 1988 issues of the *New England Journal of Medicine, Canadian Journal of Surgery, American Journal of Trauma,* and *American Journal of Psychiatry* | Gender bias is pervasive in medical research. |

| Cotton et al., 1993 | Journal | Data review | ACTG clinical trials, 1987–1990 | Women accounted for 6.7 percent of ACTG clinical trials between 1987 and 1990; women entering ACTG trials were significantly more likely to be white and less likely to have used illicit intravenous drugs than the overall population of U.S. women reported to have AIDS. The low enrollment of women in ACTG trials was influenced by demographic and geographic factors rather than attributes of specific trials There is an apparent positive influence of female research unit leadership on increasing enrollment of women in that unit's trials. |
|---|---|---|---|---|
| Meinert, 1993d | Unpublished paper | Data review | All (2,801) active proposals, proposals pending further IRB action, and proposals reviewed and completed or terminated within the last two years at the Johns Hopkins University | 181 Protocols (6.5 percent) included only males; 265 (9.5 percent) included only females; 2,355 (84 percent) included both males and females. |
| Meinert, 1993b | Unpublished paper | Data review | 293 Trials listed in the 1979 NIH inventory of clinical trials | All but 25 of the trials included both males and females; of the 25 involving only males or females, 13 involved females and 12 involved males; all 12 of the female-only trials involved uniquely or primarily female conditions, whereas only 4 of the male-only trials involved uniquely or primarily male conditions. |

*(continued)*

TABLE 2-1 Continued

| Reference | Source | Type | Coverage | Findings and Author's Conclusions |
|-----------|--------|------|----------|-----------------------------------|
| Meinert, 1993a | Unpublished paper | Literature review | All papers (38) published in the journal *Controlled Clinical Trials* since 1981 that describe an actual clinical trial | Only 28 provided explicit statements regarding gender inclusion criteria, and of these 28, only 21 provided exact counts of male and females; of the total number of subjects in these 21 trials (78,840), 72,951 were males and 5,890 were females. There is a predilection for male-based trials, at least among those authors electing to publish in this journal (or perhaps among the journal's editors). |
| NIH, National Eye Institute (NEI), 1993 | Letter to committee | Data review | Active NEI-supported clinical trials | In almost all trials, women comprise at least 40 percent of the participants; women comprise 77 percent of the subject population in trials of treatment for optic neuritis, a condition known to be more prevalent in women than men. Significant numbers of women are included in a variety of NEI-supported trials. |
| Meinert, 1993c | Unpublished paper | Data review | All (2,801) active proposals, proposals pending further IRB action, and proposals reviewed and completed or terminated within the last two years at the Johns Hopkins University | A higher percentage of male-only studies were arbitrarily male-only (75.2 percent) as opposed to female-only studies that were arbitrarily female-only (21.2 percent); however, there was a greater propensity to study females than males overall (3:1) and to study reproductive diseases (47:1) and sex-specific diseases (6:1). |
| NIH, NHLBI, 1993 | Letter to committee | Data review | All trials (49) under way at NHLBI as of May 1993 | One trial was male-only; 8 trials were female-only; women's inclusion in the remaining 40 trials ranged from 10 to 75 percent. |

| | | | | |
|---|---|---|---|---|
| Bird, 1994 | Unpublished paper | Literature review | All original articles reporting results of clinical studies in all 1990 and 1992 issues of the *Journal of the American Medical Association* (with some exceptions) | Found 207 of the 243 studies were related to gender-neutral diseases; of these, 49 percent included between one- and two-thirds women; of the remaining 51 percent, 17 percent were male-only, 6 percent were female-only, 38 percent had one-third or fewer women, and 14 percent had one-third or fewer men. Fifteen percent of single-gender studies had no apparent rationale for their single-gender design; this percentage was approximately the same for male-only and female-only studies. Female-only and male-only studies appeared to differ systematically by whether the basis of the single-gender design was disease prevalence (75 percent of female-only studies vs. 41 percent of male-only studies) or convenience (8 percent of female-only studies vs. 47 percent of male-only studies). among those studies examining gender-neutral diseases, women were more likely than men to be under-represented as research subjects. |
| NIH, National Cancer Institute (NCI), 1993 | Letter to committee | Data review | NCI-supported clinical trials active in 1992 | Of 22,483 participants in treatment trials, 12,490 were female and 9,993 were male; of 9,553 participants in prevention trials, 4,727 were female and 4,826 were male. |
| Murphy, 1993 | Journal | Data review | ACTG clinical trials, 1992 | As of August 1992, females comprised 13.2 percent of the total ACTG trial population; of adults in ACTG trials, women comprised 10.7 percent. For the 20 most recent ACTG trials with significant enrollment numbers, women comprised 15.7 percent of the trial population. |

*(continued)*

TABLE 2-1 Continued

| Reference | Source | Type | Coverage | Findings and Author's Conclusions |
|---|---|---|---|---|
| Korvick and Long, 1993 | Book chapter | Data review | ACTG clinical trials, 1986, 1992 | Representation of females in ACTG clinical trials increased from 2 percent in 1986 to over 18 percent in 1992. |
| FDA, 1993 | Government publication | Commentary | Phase I and Phase II trials | The effect of the 1977 FDA guideline regarding the participation of women of childbearing potential in clinical studies has been that women have generally not been included in Phase I nontherapeutic studies or in the earliest controlled effectiveness (Phase II) studies, except for studies of life-threatening illnesses. |
| | | Data review | 11 New drug applications (NDAs) pending in 1983 | Gender distribution of study populations generally approximated condition incidence by gender; males comprised two-thirds of the study population in studies of cardiovascular drugs (this was attributed to age group studied). |
| | | Data review | All drugs approved in 1988 (with some exceptions) | Gender distribution of study populations generally approximated condition incidence by gender; studies of two cardiovascular drugs included slightly more men than women (this was attributed to age group studied); two drugs were studied more in males for unclear reasons. |

61

| Schmucker and Vesell, 1993 | Journal | Literature and data review | All trials reported in *Clinical Pharmacology & Therapeutics* (*CP&T*) during the periods from 1969-1971, 1979-1981, and 1989-1991, and in the *British Journal of Clinical Pharmacology* (*BJCP*) during the periods 1979-1981 and 1989-1991 (with some exceptions); all drugs approved by the FDA in 1981 and 1991 that were listed in the *1992 Physician's Desk Reference* (*PDR*) | The percentage of men-only trials reported in *CP&T* increased from 27 percent to 38 percent from 1969-1971 to 1989-1991. A similar comparison in *BJCP* from 1979-1981 to 1989-1991 yielded a 5 percent increase. In both journals during these same time periods, the percentage of women-only trials declined. Of 68 clinical trials published in *CP&T* during 1991 that included both men and women, none claimed differences in drug response that were attributable to gender; the majority of trials ( > 60 percent) failed to mention whether or not the data were analyzed for gender differences. The 1992 *PDR* revealed reservations concerning use during pregnancy, but not in nonpregnant women, for nearly all drugs approved by FDA in 1981 and 1991. Despite efforts to rectify the under-representation of women as participants in clinical trials, this practice has continued during the past decade. The absence in the *PDR* of any contra-indications for drug use in nonpregnant women are difficult to interpret because they may reflect (1) no evidence of gender differences, (2) exclusion of women from test populations, or (3) failure to analyze clinical trial data for gender differences. |

*(continued)*

TABLE 2-1 Continued

| Reference | Source | Type | Coverage | Findings and Author's Conclusions |
|---|---|---|---|---|
| Elks, 1993 | Journal | Literature review | Nongonadal clinical studies reported in single volumes of three journals: *Clinical Pharmacology & Therapeutics* (*CP&T*) (January through June 1992); *American Journal of Physiology: Endocrinology and Metabolism* (*AJP*) (July through November 1992); and *Hypertension* (January through June 1992) | 49 Studies were reported in *CP&T*; 14 (29 percent) included no women and 2 (4 percent) included no men; none of these articles noted this exclusionary status in the titles. The remaining 26 studies had an average of 59 percent males. Thirty-two studies were reported in *AJP*; 10 (31 percent) included only men (one so stating in the title), 1 (3 percent) included only women, and 4 (12.5 percent) gave no statement of the gender of participants. The 16 remaining studies had an average of 57 percent males. Twenty studies were reported in *Hypertension*; 8 (40 percent) included no women (one title so stated) and 3 were large epidemiologic studies with equal representation. The 9 remaining studies had an average of 64 percent men. Frequent systematic exclusion of females has occurred; even in both-sex studies, more men than women are included than would be likely by chance. |

| Zahm et al., In press | Unpublished paper | Literature review | Cancer epidemiologic studies published between 1971 and 1990 in *American Journal of Epidemiology, American Journal of Industrial Medicine, Archives of Environmental Health, British Journal of Industrial Medicine, International Journal of Epidemiology, Journal of the National Cancer Institute, Journal of Occupational Medicine,* and *Scandinavian Journal of Work, Environment, and Health* | Of a total of 1,233 studies, 562 (46 percent) included only white men, while the remaining 671 studies (54 percent) included subjects from other race-gender groups. Of these, 35 percent included white women, but only 14 percent presented any analyses of the white women specifically. The proportions with analyses of non-white women (any: 2 percent; detailed: 1 percent) or non-white men (any: 7 percent; detailed: 3 percent) were also small. Studies with detailed analyses of women and minorities tended to use weaker methodologies (i.e., proportionate mortality or cross-sectional design) than the studies of white men and were less able to provide convincing data on the occupational cancer risks of women and minorities. |

NOTE: ADAMHA = Alcohol, Drug Abuse, and Mental Health Administration; CDC = Centers for Disease Control and Prevention; FDA = Food and Drug Administration; GAO = General Accounting Office; IOM = Institute of Medicine; IRB = Institutional Review Board; NIH = National Institutes of Health; NOW = National Organization for Women; and PMA = Pharmaceutical Manufacturers Association.

ate. Concern also has been expressed about the possibility that what is known about the natural history of the diseases and their treatment in men is inapplicable to women. Recent research efforts, however, have begun to address these concerns.

## Heart Disease

Every year 2.5 million American women are hospitalized for heart disease (Wenger et al., 1993). Of this number, 500,000 die, half of them (approximately 250,000) from coronary heart disease (CHD) (Field, 1993). CHD is the single most frequent cause of death among women. Yet despite these compelling statistics, a perception persists among the public and physicians that women do not contract heart disease as often as men, and that when they do, it is not as serious.

Part of this perception is based on results obtained by the Framingham study, a longitudinal study launched in 1948 that followed a cohort of male and female subjects between the ages of 36 and 68 over a period of 12 years. It found that mortality rates for CHD were much higher among men than women—approximately three male deaths for every female death. Based on the results from this and other studies, males in their middle years appeared to be especially vulnerable to CHD; women were assumed to be relatively protected from this disease.

It has since been shown that women are not protected from CHD, but rather that they develop the disease (and die from it) later in life. Rates of heart disease increase gradually in postmenopausal women until they begin to manifest myocardial infarction (MI) at the same rate as men. There is evidence to suggest that this increase is caused by the loss of the protective effect of estrogen, and that hormone replacement therapy might restore this protective factor (Fackelmann, 1993). Estrogen replacement therapy in postmenopausal women, however, has produced mixed results.

Coronary events are rare in women under age 65: women in the 75-84 age group exhibit a significantly higher rate of CHD than women in the 35-44 age group (NHLBI, 1990). Moreover, women comprise 59 percent of the population over age 65 and 64 percent of the population over age 74; there are 182 women for every 100 men over 75 years of age (Gurwitz et al., 1992). Thus, a failure to include people over 65 in clinical studies of heart disease has serious ramifications for women, who develop the disease later than men and are 20 years older at their first MI. It suggests that women's manifestations of heart disease may not have been adequately studied.

The major identified risk factors for heart disease (including hypertension, cigarette smoking, and obesity) are reliable predictors for both men and women, but men and women differ in their manifestations of CHD. For men the most common initial manifestation is MI, but for women it is uncomplicated angina pectoris (Wenger et al., 1993). For example, 69 percent of the women but only 30 percent of the men in the Framingham study had angina pectoris as their initial manifestation of CHD (NIH, 1990). In addition, women may continue to have angina for a number of years without experiencing an MI. Thus, angina pectoris came to be viewed as relatively benign: even though it was the most common manifestation of CHD for women, it was not as widespread or as immediate in its effects as MI was for men. This provided yet another reason for regarding CHD as fatal primarily for men, and not for women, despite the fact that some evidence from the Framingham study indicates that an initial MI is more likely to be fatal in women than in men (NIH, 1990).

Several well-known studies of cardiovascular disease have not included any women participants. These include the MRFIT, the Coronary Drug Project (CDP), Lipid Research Clinic, and the Physicians' Health Study, all of which have had widespread influence on the treatment and prevention of heart disease (Healy, 1991). MRFIT was a study of 12,866 men between the ages of 35 and 57, designed to assess the efficacy of intervention for individuals at high risk for coronary heart disease because of elevated serum lipids, hypertension, and cigarette smoking (Multiple Risk Factor Intervention Trial Research Group, 1977). CDP was a randomized, controlled clinical trial designed to evaluate the efficacy of several different lipid-influencing drugs in prolonging the lives of men (age 30 through 64 at entry) with a prior history of myocardial infarction (Meinert, 1986). The Physicians' Health Study was a randomized controlled trial of 22,071 male physicians designed to determine whether low-dose aspirin therapy decreases the risk of myocardial infarction and whether beta-carotene reduces the risk of cancer (Steering Committee of the Physicians' Health Study Research Group, 1989).

Because these studies did not include women, they could not produce definitive information about prevention and treatment of heart disease in women. Critics have claimed that the extrapolation to women of the male-generated findings of MRFIT, CDP, and PHS is potentially faulty because it ignores the importance of estrogen in women as an antiatherogenic agent (Healy, 1991) and because the natural history of CHD is different in men and women. They have also claimed that such gender-exclusive research reinforces the myth that cardiovascular disease is a uniquely male affliction (Healy, 1991), when cardiovascular disease is the leading cause of death in both women and men.

Those who defend the male-only design of MRFIT, CDP, and the Physicians' Health Study point to the epidemiology of heart disease at the time the studies were initiated: a perceived epidemic of heart disease among middle-aged men explains the studies' focus on males. The failure to detect the actual rate of heart disease in women may have resulted from gender bias; recent studies show evidence of a sex bias in the management of coronary heart disease (Ayanian and Epstein, 1991; Steingart et al., 1991). The age differential may also have played a role in women's exclusion—women are typically affected by heart disease 10 to 15 years later than men. Recruiting older persons, male or female, complicates recruitment strategies (that is, required recruitment at large numbers of retirement communities as well as major medical centers) and poses a challenge to retention of subjects (as a result of comorbid conditions, for example). It is also conceivable, however, that age bias played a primary role in the male-only design of the studies.

## AIDS

AIDS research is another area in which claims have been made that women and women's health interests have been understudied. When the scientific community first became aware of AIDS in 1981, it was considered a disease of homosexual men, and indeed the absolute number of cases of AIDS in men continues to be greater than the absolute number of cases in women. Nevertheless, the first cases of AIDS in women were reported in 1981, and the number of cases in women has been increasing rapidly since 1986. The response of the federal research enterprise has not kept pace with the spread of the disease among women; only now, in 1994, are comprehensive studies looking at the epidemiology of the disease in women.

The delay in examining how AIDS manifests itself in women has resulted in women's conditions being conspicuously absent from the list of conditions defined by the Centers for Disease Control and Prevention (CDC) to constitute AIDS, and this in turn has resulted in the denial of benefit and treatment programs to women. Finally, in clinical trials of AIDS drugs, which often may provide significant sources of first-rate medical care and access to experimental treatments for persons with AIDS, the numbers of women participating lags behind expectations for a disease that is increasing the most rapidly among women.

Perhaps more important, where women have been the focus of clinical research the primary research question has been how to reduce or prevent a vertical transmission of human immunodeficiency virus (HIV) from a pregnant woman to a fetus or newborn, not how to treat the female-specific manifestations of HIV diseases. Moreover, until very recently there has been almost no research explaining the mechanisms of male-to-female transmission of HIV and little research directed at the development of anti-viricidal preparations that could be used by women to reduce their chances of contracting the infection through sexual activity (Faden et al., in press).

## Women of Childbearing Age in Early Phases of Drug Trials

The FDA recently revised its policy on the exclusion of women of childbearing potential from early phases of drug trials (FDA, 1993). The 1977 guideline had recommended that a "woman of childbearing potential" be excluded from Phase I and early Phase II drug trials except under limited circumstances, for example, when the use of an investigational drug was considered to be a life-saving or life-prolonging measure, such as cancer therapies, and, more recently, AIDS therapies. The guideline broadly defined a woman of childbearing potential as a "premenopausal female capable of becoming pregnant" (FDA, 1977). Included in the definition were women on oral, injectable, or mechanical contraception; women who were "single"; and women whose partners had been vasectomized or were using mechanical contraception. Women prisoners could be excluded from the guideline's restriction because they were "not in the appropriate environment to become pregnant" during a study. (See Chapter 6.)

FDA concluded that the guidelines have limited the collection of drug response information that would have been useful in designing later phases of trials and may have slowed detection of gender-related variations in drug effects (FDA, 1993a). As a result, FDA issued a revised guideline in July 1993 describing the earlier restriction as an "unnecessary Federal impediment to the inclusion of women in the earliest stages of drug development" (FDA, 1993b). As currently written, the 1993 guideline does not now *mandate* the inclusion of women of childbearing potential, or women in general, in particular types of trials, relying instead on the "interplay of ethical, social, medical, legal and political forces" to encourage greater participation of women in the earlier stages of clinical trials (FDA, 1993b). It is unclear how this change in FDA guidelines will change the behavior of those performing trials.

## Clinical Trial Registries

The inability of the committee to draw conclusions from available data underscores the need for systematized collection of information by, at the very least, all federal agencies that conduct or support research involving human subjects. While these sorts of efforts have been undertaken in the past, they have not been wholly successful or enduring.

In 1974 NIH established a centralized registry of NIH-funded clinical trials that operated for almost five years before it was abandoned in 1979 as a cost-saving measure (Dickersin and Min, 1993). In 1985 the registry was reestablished in NIH Office of Medical Applications of Research (OMAR) in response to a need for a single source of information on clinical trials, as well as to assist in responding to reporting requirements of the Stephenson-

Wydler Technology Innovation Act of 1980[2] (NIH, 1992a). For two reasons, however, the information contained in the OMAR registry is not considered to be complete: (1) reporting of clinical studies is not mandatory, and (2) it was not until 1988 that the registry began collecting data on the gender of study participants, data that is not yet available in aggregate form. Strategies for redesigning the OMAR registry so that it is more accessible to researchers who want to submit data and to others who want to extract data are currently being explored (personal communication with J. Ferguson, OMAR Director, August 1993).

The NIH Revitalization Act of 1993, passed in June 1993, promises to enhance the availability of information about women's participation in clinical studies. One provision of the act requires the directors of NIH, ORWH, and the National Library of Medicine (NLM) to collaborate in establishing a "data system for the collection, storage, analysis, retrieval, and dissemination of information regarding research on women's health that is conducted or supported by the national research institutes." The act also requires that the data system include a registry of clinical trials of experimental treatments that have been developed for research on women's health, as well as information about subject eligibility criteria, gender, race, ethnicity, age, and the location of the trial site(s). The act also stipulates that principal investigators of clinical trials provide this information to the registry within 30 days after it is available, and, once a trial is completed, provide the registry with information about the results, including potential toxicities or adverse effects associated with the treatments evaluated. At the time of this writing, a conference on future strategies for clinical study registration was being planned by NIH.

There are numerous clinical trial registries throughout the world. Most of these are focused on specific medical conditions, such as AIDS or cancer, or on specific fields of medicine, such a neurosurgery or perinatology. An ongoing University of Maryland project to identify clinical trial registries around the world counted 27 registries in existence as of June, 1992 (Dickersin and Garcia-Lopez, 1992). The goals of the project are to provide information to researchers and interested parties and to form an international network of registers.

## CONCLUSIONS AND RECOMMENDATIONS

Over the past 50 years the scientific and political communities have grappled with the question of just how far they should go in protecting the human subjects of medical research, especially pregnant women. Reaction to the atrocities of the Nazis was reinforced by further abuses in the 1960s and 1970s and by the tragedies of thalidomide and DES. Early federal policies and regulations in this area were stringent and protectionist, grouping pregnant women with other "vulnerable" populations—children, prisoners, and the mentally impaired. Following the example of AIDS activists, however, women's health groups have successfully lobbied for changes that encourage and, more recently, require investigators to include an "appropriate" number of women in their study populations.

The pendulum now appears to be swinging toward the "inclusionist" side of the argument, where a consensus seems to be emerging in the scientific and political communities, and among the general public as well. Other chapters of this report review the ethical and scientific arguments that bolster this consensus, as well as the social and legal issues it raises. The committee, however, has identified an important underlying consideration: the lack of reliable, comprehensive information on the actual participation of women and various subgroups of women in clinical studies, today or in the past.

Information on gender, racial, and ethnic composition of study populations is not currently available in any accessible form. The NIH Revitalization Act's mandate that ORWH create a registry focused solely on women's health and the collection of women's health data is too narrow—without information on men's health issues and men's levels of participation in such studies, monitoring of the relative levels of participation in the future will be difficult and open to bias.

**The committee supports the efforts of NIH to establish a registry of clinical studies and recommends that such a registry include information on the participation of women and men and on the racial and ethnic composition of participants in such studies, as well as the research questions addressed, that such information be reasonably accessible to investigators and the public, and that the scope of the studies included in the registry be comprehensive.**

The committee views this registry as a potentially valuable resource in the development of national research agendas, preparation of reports to Congress, preparation of grant requests by investigators, recruitment of study participants, and development of cooperative efforts among institutes and other study sponsors, including multicenter studies. Such a registry would facilitate the development of the NIH research agenda. Another purpose might be to provide data for reporting to Congress on implementation of the legislative mandate to include women and racial and ethnic groups in clinical studies.

A comprehensive scope (i.e., who is required to report to whom and what is required to be reported to the registry) is vital to achieving the above purposes and avoiding the potential waste of limited research dollars on duplicative research. At a minimum, the registry should include ongoing studies as well as published studies.

**The committee recommends that NIH work with other federal agencies and departments that conduct clinical research to ensure reporting of all federally funded clinical studies. The committee further recommends that representatives of NIH initiate discussions with FDA concerning the feasibility of including privately funded studies in such a registry.**

The kinds of information to be included and reported to the registry should be uniform. In addition to gender composition of the study population, the registry might include an abstract of the study, the investigator name, and other study population characteristics, such as age and racial and ethnic identification. The committee proposes in Chapter 8 that this information be collected by IRBs; the current legislation concerning the establishment of a clinical trials registry for women's health proposes that such information be collected by investigators.

In implementating such a registry, NIH should consider the costs, reporting pathways, accessibility of information, enforceability of reporting requirements, and quality control. NIH should also consider and take precautions against problems that might be posed by such a registry, particularly with private industry involvement, including considerations of confidentiality, insurance reimbursement implications, endorsement of studies through inclusion in registry, access to non-peer-reviewed studies, administrative burden, and cost considerations.

## NOTES

1.  The three institutes that comprised ADAMHA—the National Institute of Mental Health (NIMH), the National Institute of Drug Abuse (NIDA), and the National Institute of Alcoholism and Alcohol Abuse (NIAAA)—were joined, in their capacity as research institutions, with the NIH in October, 1992. The service components of ADAMHA now operate under the name of Substance Abuse and Mental Health Services Administration.

2.  The Stephenson-Wydler Technology Innovation Act of 1980 called for efforts to "ensure the full use of the results of the nation's federal investment in research and development." One section of the act specifies that "each federal agency which operates or directs one or more federal laboratories shall prepare biennially a report summarizing the activities performed by that agency and its Federal laboratories."

# REFERENCES

AMA (American Medical Association) Council on Ethical and Judicial Affairs. 1991. Gender disparities in clinical decision making. *Journal of the American Medical Association* 266(4):559-562.

AMA. 1991. Women in Medicine in America: In the Mainstream. Chicago: AMA.

Auerbach, J.D. 1993. The emergence of the women's health research agenda: Some preliminary analysis. Draft revision of a paper presented at the annual meeting of the Association for Public Policy Analysis and Management, Denver, Colo., October 29-31, 1992.

Ayanian, J.Z., and Epstein, A.M. 1991. Differences in the use of procedures between women and men hospitalized for coronary heart disease. *New England Journal of Medicine* 325(4):221-225.

Beecher, H.K. 1966. Ethics and clinical research. *New England Journal of Medicine* 274:1354-1360.

Bird, C.E. 1994. Women's representation as subjects in clinical studies: A pilot study of research published in *JAMA* in 1990 and 1992. In: Women and Health Research: Ethical and Legal Issues of Including Women in Clinical Studies, Volume 2, A. Mastroianni, R. Faden, and D. Federman, eds. Washington, D.C.: National Academy Press.

Boston Women's Health Book Collective. 1973. Our Bodies, Ourselves. New York: Simon and Schuster.

Charo, R.A. 1992. Memo to Human Subjects Committee re: Frequency of exclusion of fertile women from drug studies (University of Wisconsin Experience, 1989-1990). 23 March.

Christie, G.A. 1962. Thalidomide and congenital abnormalities. *Lancet* 2:249.

Cotton, D.J., He, W.L., Feinberg, J., and Finkelstein, D.M. 1993. Determinants of accrual of women to a large, multicenter HIV/AIDS clinical trials program in the United States. *Journal of Acquired Immune Deficiency* 6:1322-1328.

Cotton, P. 1990a. Examples abound of gaps in medical knowledge because of groups excluded from scientific study. *Journal of the American Medical Association* 263(8):1052.

Cotton, P. 1990b. Is there still too much extrapolation from data on middle-aged white men? *Journal of the American Medical Association* 263(8):1049-1050.

Cotton, P. 1992. Women's Health Initiative leads way as research begins to fill gender gaps. *Journal of the American Medical Association* 267(4):469-473.

Dickersin, K., and Garcia-Lopez, F. 1992. Keeping posted: Regulatory process effects clinical trial registration in Spain. *Controlled Clinical Trials* 13:507-512.

Dickersin, K., and Min, Y.-I. 1993. NIH clinical trials and publication bias. *Online Journal of Current Clinical Trials* (28 April), Doc. No. 50.

Dresser, R. 1992. Wanted: single, white male for medical research. *Hastings Center Report* (Jan/Feb):24-29.

Edwards, L.D. 1991. Most major companies test medicines in women, monitor data for gender differences. In: In Development: New Medicines for Women. Washington, D.C.: Pharmaceutical Manufacturers Association.

Eichler, M., Reisman, A.L., and Borins, E. 1992. Gender bias in medical research. *Women and Therapy—A Feminist Quarterly* 12(4):61-71.

Elks, M.L. 1993. The right to participate in research studies. *Journal of Laboratory and Clinical Medicine* 122(2):130-136.

Fackelmann, K.A. 1993. Heart findings support hormonal therapy. *Science News* 143(16):246.

Faden, R.R., and Beauchamp, T.L. 1986. A History and Theory of Informed Consent. New York: Oxford University Press.

Faden, R.R., Kass, N., and McGraw, D. In press. Women as vessels and vectors: Lessons from the HIV epidemic. In: Feminism and Bioethics: Beyond Reproduction, S. Wolf, ed. New York: Oxford University Press.

FDA (Food and Drug Administration). 1977. General Consideration for the Clinical Evaluation of Drugs. Rockville, Md.: FDA.

FDA. 1993. Guideline for the Study and Evaluation of Gender Differences in the Clinical Evaluation of Drugs; Notice. *Federal Register* 58(139):39406-39416.

FDA. 1992. Statement: Women in Clinical Trials. 29 October. Rockville, Md.: FDA.

Field, M. 1993. Heart disease, estrogen focus of major study. *Johns Hopkins University Gazette* 22(21):1-3.

Gannon, L., Luchetta, T., Rhodes, K., Pardie, L., and Segrist, D. 1992. Sex bias in psychological research: Progress or complacency? *American Psychologist* (March):389-396.

GAO (General Accounting Office). 1990. Summary of testimony by Mark V. Nadel on problems in implementing the National Institutes of Health Policy on Women in Study Populations. Given before the Subcommittee on Health and the Environment, Committee on Energy and Commerce, House of Representatives, 18 June. Washington, D.C.: GAO.

GAO. 1992. Women's Health; FDA Needs to Ensure More Study of Gender Differences in Prescription Drug Testing. GAO/HRD-93-17. Washington, D.C.: GAO.

Gurwitz, G.H., Col, N.F, and Avorn, J. 1992. The exclusion of the elderly and women from clinical trials in acute myocardial infarction. *Journal of the American Medical Association* 268(11):1417-1422.

Healy, B. 1991. The Yentl syndrome. *New England Journal of Medicine* 325(4):274-276.

Herman, R. 1992. What doctors don't know about women: NIH tries to close the gender gap in research. *Washington Post*, 8 December (Health Section):10.

Hooper, C. 1990. Some drug trials show gender bias. *Journal of NIH Research* 2:47-48.

IOM (Institute of Medicine). 1991a. Assessing Future Research Needs: Mental and Addictive Disorders in Women. Washington, D.C.: National Academy Press.

IOM. 1991b. Issues in the Inclusion of Women in Clinical Trials. Report of a Planning Panel of the Institute of Medicine's Division of Health Sciences Policy, 1-2 March. Washington, D.C.: National Academy Press.

Johnson, T. 1992. Health research that excludes women is bad science. *Chronicle of Higher Education* (14 October):B1.

Johnson, T., and Fee, E. 1994. Women's participation in clinical research: From protectionism to access. In: Women and Health Research: Ethical and Legal Issues of Including Women in Clinical Studies, Volume 2, A. Mastroianni, R. Faden, and D. Federman, eds. Washington, D.C.: National Academy Press.

Jones, J.H. 1981. Bad Blood. New York: Free Press.

King, P.A. 1992. The dangers of difference. *Hastings Center Report* 22(6):35-38.

Kinney, E.L., Trautmann, J., Gold, J.A., Vesell, E.S., and Zelis, R. 1981. Underrepresentation of women in new drug trials. *Annals of Internal Medicine* 95(4):495-499.

Kolata, G. 1990. NIH neglects women, study says. *New York Times* 19 June:B11, C6.

Korvick, J.A., and Long, I.L. 1993. Update on clinical trials and pharmaceutical regimens for women with HIV infection. In: Until the Cure: Caregiving for Women with HIV, A. Kurth, ed. New Haven: Yale University Press.

Larson, E. In press. Exclusion of certain groups from clinical research. *Image: Journal of Nursing Scholarship*.

Levey, B.A. 1991. Bridging the gender gap in research. *Clinical Pharmacology and Therapeutics* 50:641-646.

Levi, J. 1991. Unproven AIDS therapies: The Food and Drug Administration and ddI. Pp. 9-37 in *Biomedical Politics*, K. Hanna, ed. Washington, D.C.: National Academy Press.

Levine, C. 1993. Women as research subjects: New priorities, new questions. In: Emerging Issues in Biomedical Policy: An Annual Review, Volume 2, R.H. Blank and A.L. Bonnicksen, eds. New York: Columbia University Press.

Long, I.L. 1993. Women's access to government-sponsored AIDS/HIV clinical trials: Status report, critique and recommendations. 26 March. Unpublished manuscript.

McGuire, P. 1993. Let's stop guessing about women's health. *New York Times,* 2 March (Editorial).

Meinert, C.L. 1986. Clinical Trials: Design, Conduct, and Analysis. New York: Oxford University Press.

Meinert, C.L. 1993a. Memo to co-chairs of IOM Committee on the Legal and Ethical Issues Relating to the Inclusion of Women in Clinical Studies, 5 May. Re: Clinical Trials in Controlled Clinical Trials.

Meinert, C.L. 1993b. Memo to co-chairs of IOM Committee on the Legal and Ethical Issues Relating to the Inclusion of Women in Clinical Studies, 5 May. Re: NIH Inventory of Clinical Trials.

Meinert, C.L. 1993c. Memo to co-chairs of IOM Committee on Legal and Ethical Issues Relating to the Inclusion of Women in Clinical Studies, 21 May. Re: On Gender Coverage at Johns Hopkins University.

Meinert, C.L. 1993d. Memo to co-chairs of IOM Committee on Legal and Ethical Issues Relating to the Inclusion of Women in Clinical Studies, 14 April. Re: Johns Hopkins University IRB Counts.

Multiple Risk-Factor Intervention Trial Group. 1977. Statistical design considerations in the NHLI multiple risk factor intervention trial (MRFIT). *Journal of Chronic Diseases* 30:261-275.

Murphy, D. 1993. Women in clinical trials: HIV-infected women. *Food and Drug Law Journal* 48(2):175-179.

National Commission (National Commission for the Protection of Human Subjects of Biomedical and Behavioral Research). 1978. The Belmont Report: Ethical Principles and Guidelines for the Protection of Human Subjects of Research. Washington, D.C.: Government Printing Office.

NIH (National Institutes of Health). 1992a. National Institutes of Health Clinical Trials Report, FY 1988-FY 1989 (Office of Medical Applications of Research). Bethesda, Md.

NIH. 1992b. Opportunities for Research on Women's Health. Report of a conference, September 4-6, 1991, Hunt Valley, Maryland. NIH Publication No. 92-3457. Bethesda, Md.

NIH, National Cancer Institute. 1993. Letter to Anna Mastroianni from Iris J. Schneider Re: inclusion of males and females in clinical trials supported by the National Cancer Institute in FY 1992 (23 June).

NIH, National Eye Institute. 1993. Letter to Curtis Meinert from Richard Mowery (Director, Division of Collaborative Clinical Research) regarding Dr. Meinert's request for data about clinical trials (20 May).

NIH, National Heart, Lung, and Blood Institute. 1990. Women's Health Issues. A presentation at the 159th meeting of the National Heart, Lung, and Blood Advisory Council (6 September), Bethesda, Md.

NIH, National Heart, Lung, and Blood Institute. 1993. Letter to Curt Meinert Re: Clinical Trials Performed by the NHLBI (26 May).

NOW Legal Defense and Education Fund. 1993. Citizens' petition. Petition proposing change in FDA policy of encouraging private drug companies to exclude nonsterilized women from their experimental drug trials.

Okie, S. 1990. NIH slow to include women in disease research. *Washington Post,* 19 June:A10.

Pham, H., Freeman, P., and Kohn, N. 1992. Understanding the Second Epidemic: The Status of Research on Women and AIDS in the United States. Washington, D.C.: Center for Women's Policy Studies.

PMA (Pharmaceutical Manufacturers Association). 1991. In Development: New Medicines for Women. Survey of 263 new medicines in testing for use in women. Washington, D.C.: PMA.

PMA. 1992a. In Development: AIDS Medicines, Drugs, and Vaccines. 1992 Survey Report: 91 Medicines in Testing, 3 Approved this Past Year. Washington, D.C.: PMA.

PMA. 1992b. Women in AIDS and orphan drug trials. *Pharmaceutical Manufacturers Association Newsletter* 34(42):3.

Prescott, S. 1978. Why researchers don't study women: The responses of 62 researchers. *Sex Roles* 4(6):899-905.

Reardon, P., and Prescott, S. 1977. Sex as reported in a recent sample of psychological research. *Psychology of Women Quarterly* 2(2):157-160.

Rothman, D.J., and Edgar, H. 1990. New rules for new drugs: The challenge of AIDS to the regulatory process. *Milbank Quarterly Supplement.* 68(1):111-142.

Rothman, D.J., and Edgar, H. 1992. Scientific Rigor and Medical Realities: Placebo Trials in Cancer and AIDS Research. Pp. 194-206 in AIDS: The Making of a Chronic Disease, E. Fee and D. M. Fox, eds. Berkeley: University of California Press.

Schmucker, D.L., and Vesell, E.S. 1993. Underrepresentation of women in clinical drug trials. *Clinical Pharmacology and Therapeutics* 54:11-15.

Sherman, S.S. 1993. Gender, health, and responsible research. *Clinics in Geriatric Medicine* 9(1):261-269.

Steering Committee of the Physicians' Health Study Research Group. 1989. Final report on the aspirin component of the ongoing physicians' health study. *New England Journal of Medicine* 321(3):129-135.

Steingart, R.M., Packer, M., Hamm, P., Coglianese, M.E., Gersh, B., Geltman, E.M., et al. 1991. Sex differences in the management of coronary artery disease. *New England Journal of Medicine* 325(4):226-230.

Stevens, C. 1992. How women get bad medicine. *Washingtonian* (June):75-77, 94-98.

USDHEW (U.S. Department of Health, Education, and Welfare). 1973. Final Report of the Tuskegee Syphilis Study Ad Hoc Advisory Panel. Washington, D.C.

USPHS (U.S. Public Health Service). 1985. Report of the Public Health Service Task Force on Women's Health Issues. *Public Health Reports* 100(1):73-106.

Ungerleider, R.S., and Friedman, M.A. 1991. Sex, trials, and datatapes. *Journal of the National Cancer Institute* 83(1):16-17.

Wenger, N.K., Speroff, L., and Packard, B. 1993. Cardiovascular health and disease in women. *New England Journal of Medicine* 329(4):247-256.

Williams, K., and Manace Borins, E.F. 1993. Gender bias in a peer-reviewed medical journal. *Journal of the American Medical Women's Association* 48(5):160-162.

Zahm, S.H., Pottern, L.M., Lewis, D.R., Ward, M.H., and White, D.W. In press. Inclusion of women and minorities in occupational cancer epidemiological research. *Journal of Occupational Medicine.*

# 3

# Justice in Clinical Studies:
# Guiding Principles

## CONCEPTIONS OF JUSTICE

Concerns about justice in the conduct of biomedical research involving human subjects received little attention until the publication of the *Belmont Report* (National Commission for the Protection of Human Subjects of Biomedical and Behavioral Research, 1978). In that document, the National Commission for the Protection of Human Subjects of Biomedical and Behavioral Research (National Commission) outlined three ethical principles that should govern research:

1. *Respect for persons* reflects two basic convictions: "first, that individuals should be treated as autonomous agents, and second, that persons with diminished autonomy are entitled to protection."
2. *Beneficence* is understood as the obligation to maximize possible benefits and minimize possible harms in conducting research.
3. *Justice*, the third of these basic principles, is the main focus of this chapter.

The *Belmont Report* states that "injustice arises from social, racial, sexual and cultural biases institutionalized in society." Women as a class were not the primary concern of the National Commission's work. In sketching the historical background related to justice in research, its report cited the following examples of injustices:

During the 19th and early 20th centuries the burdens of serving as research subjects fell largely upon poor ward patients, while the benefits of improved medical care flowed primarily to private patients. Subsequently, the exploitation of unwilling prisoners as research subjects in Nazi concentration camps was condemned as a particularly flagrant injustice. In this country, in the 1940s, the Tuskegee syphilis study used disadvantaged, rural black men to study the untreated course of a disease that is by no means confined to that population. These subjects were deprived of demonstrably effective treatment in order not to interrupt the project, long after such treatment became available.

The conception of justice embodied in the *Belmont Report* is essentially that of *distributive justice,* a notion pertinent to situations that call for the fair allocation of society's benefits and burdens. Other conceptions of justice may apply in differing situations. For example, *procedural justice* applies to a wide variety of social, legal, and institutional matters in which achieving a fair or unbiased result is dependent on adherence to a set of well-ordered procedures, such as the legal requirements of due process. The notion of *compensatory justice* goes beyond that of fairness in distribution in an attempt to remedy or redress past wrongs. An example from the history of human subjects research is that of monetary payments made to survivors of the Tuskegee syphilis study or to their relatives, to compensate them for the harm or wrong done by the study.

## The Distributive Paradigm

Of these conceptions of justice, the most widely applicable to human subjects research is *distributive justice.* Clinical studies, especially those in the earliest stages where safety or toxicity is being measured, often involve substantial risks to human subjects. Those risks should be allocated fairly. It is impossible to arrive at a precise *general* definition of fair allocation, however, because the criteria for fairness may differ from one context to another. Some situations require an *equal* distribution (for example, one person, one vote), while others call for an *equitable* distribution (such as from each according to ability, to each according to need). The precise definition of fairness in allocation is determined by the context.

In the context of clinical studies, fair allocation is best characterized as equity. That is, because research carries both benefits and burdens, fairness requires that no one group—gender, racial, ethnic, or socioeconomic group— receive disproportionate benefits or bear disproportionate burdens of research. It is not readily apparent, however, what is to count as "proportionate" or "disproportionate" benefits and burdens.

If justice requires an appropriate representation of women in the conduct of clinical studies, there remains the problem of elucidating what is to count as "appropriate representation." Does it mean that women should be included in research in numbers equal to their representation in the population as a whole? Should it be viewed as including women in proportion to their representation among those afflicted by the disease or condition in question? Or does it mean that the research results should pertain equally to all afflicted groups, and hence that the research population must be constructed to assure appropriate analyses for providing this information? This difficulty in defining the kind of representation required by distributive justice influenced the committee's consideration of issues relating to the composition of study populations (see Chapter 4).

It should be emphasized that the general concept of distributive justice, and thus the principle of appropriate representation, applies to classes of people rather than to individuals. Therefore, it would not be a violation of the principle of justice if particular individuals in a class were not recruited as research subjects. Only if the benefits or burdens of research are found to accrue systematically to specified classes of people to the exclusion of other classes would the research violate the principle of distributive justice.

One aspect of justice in research is thus the requirement of a "fitting" match: the population from which research subjects are drawn should reflect the population to be served by the actual or projected results of the research. The chief concern over the past several decades has been that some groups, such as incarcerated men, have been "overstudied." The *Belmont Report* addressed this concern by urging that:

> The selection of research subjects needs to be scrutinized in order to determine whether some classes (e.g., welfare patients, particular racial and ethnic minorities, or persons confined to institutions) are being systematically selected simply because of their easy availability, their compromised position, or their manipulability, rather than for reasons directly related to the problem being studied.

More recently, attention has turned away from the problem of unduly subjecting certain groups to disproportionate risks and toward the problem of denying the benefits of research to certain classes of people who have not frequently been the subjects of research. This observation has been made with regard to heart disease in women (see Chapter 2), but the same concern applies to subgroups of women such as women of color, diverse ethnic groups, and older women. For the overall biomedical research agenda to comply with the requirements of justice, studies must not only include women as well as men, but also women and men from different age cohorts and different racial and ethnic groups. If clinical studies are intended to benefit the population as a whole, then the systematic exclusion of women from such studies places them at an unfair disadvantage.

Conversely, justice also demands that (in the words of the *Belmont*

*Report*) "research should not unduly involve persons from groups unlikely to be among the beneficiaries of subsequent applications of the research." This requirement pertains not so much to women in general as to poor women and women of racial and ethnic groups. The same holds true for U.S.-sponsored research conducted in other countries. If people in developing countries are recruited as participants in research, two conditions must be fulfilled to meet the requirements of the distributive conception of justice:

1.   The design and determination of acceptable risk-benefit ratios must be evaluated with the same standards as when such research is carried out in the United States.
2.   Beneficiaries of the research outcomes must include people in the developing countries where the research is conducted, as well as in the United States.

In short, justice is to be construed as a universal requirement, not confined within the borders of any one nation.

### Application to Clinical Studies

According to the basic conception of distributive justice, a categorical exclusion of women from clinical studies would surely violate the principle of justice. But even when women are not categorically excluded, justice may still be violated in particular research programs or in the overall national research agenda. This violation of justice can take several different forms. First, studies of diseases or conditions that affect both genders but that have included a disproportionately small number of people of one gender are presumptively unjust (an example is that of heart disease, as noted above). Second, some conditions or diseases that affect only or primarily one gender have received far less research attention than the numbers of people affected would appear to warrant. An example commonly put forward for women is that of menopause; another is the manifestations of human immunodeficiency virus (HIV) disease in women (see Chapter 2). An example that applies to men is the study of functional impotence in older men. Another long-standing failure to meet the requirements of justice has been the exclusion from certain drug studies of women "of childbearing potential," a category broadly construed to include the vast majority of women for a substantial portion of their lives.

What are the consequences of violating the principles of justice when conducting clinical studies? Exclusion or underrepresentation affects both women during the time they are denied access to studies and women who receive the treatment that was under investigation following the completion of clinical studies. In the most general sense, the failure to match study groups with target user groups can cause the unstudied or understudied group to receive no medical treatment, ineffective treatment, or even harmful treatment. If the drug has not been tested at all on pregnant or lactating women during the research phase, for example, then information is lacking about the safety and efficacy of the drug for the women themselves, as well as for the fetus. This may result in undertreatment of pregnant or lactating women until postapproval studies are available.

Even when some data are collected about women's responses to a particular treatment—including pregnant and lactating women—information may still be lacking about how a proposed treatment will affect specific subgroups of women with clinically relevant characteristics, such as women who have disabilities or are elderly or poor. According to the traditional conception of distributive justice, this sort of discrimination is unjust and may have the consequence of providing less effective health care for some women than for comparable men because the knowledge base that guides health care practices is unfairly skewed.

Under the distributive paradigm, what steps might be required to remedy the injustice of excluding women from clinical studies? The minimum measure required is the appropriate inclusion of women in future clinical studies, as described above. According to the mainstream conception of distributive justice, current inequities are to be rectified by abandoning policies or practices that have deliberately or unwittingly excluded women from the study of diseases or disorders that afflict both men and women. Beyond that step, however, other views may come into play.

## Justice and the Research Agenda: Oppression and Power

The distributive paradigm is not the only conception of justice, despite its preeminence in the *Belmont Report* and ensuing literature. For example, Iris Marion Young and other writers presenting a feminist view have argued that *oppression* qualifies as a concern of justice, and that some important aspects of oppression are not purely matters of distribution (Young, 1990). These scholars have argued that it is not random or accidental that women are disadvantaged in this way, but rather a result and further dimension of women's generally oppressed status in society.

For example, the research agenda has historically neglected many important questions regarding women's health needs, yet there has been a substantial body of research directed at gaining control over women's reproductive capacity (Sherwin, 1994). This concentration on women's reproductive role not only assumes the conventional view that women are, by nature, to be responsible and available for reproductive activities; it has the further consequence of legitimizing, reinforcing, and further entrenching such views and the attitudes that accompany them. This feminist critique also explains what some contend is a corresponding lack of attention to problems of peri- and postmenopausal women as topics of research.

There are other consequences that flow from this broader conception of justice. One of the reasons that women traditionally have been excluded from clinical studies of conditions that affect both men and women is that "their hormonal fluctuations 'confound' or 'confuse' research results" (DeBruin, 1994). Acceptance of the view that men are the norm, and women deviant or problematic for the conduct of biomedical research, serves to perpetuate the practice of excluding women so that the scientific results of studies are not "confounded" (see discussion of *male norm* in Chapter 5).

According to this view, remedies for past injustices would require paying special attention to women in the research agenda. To some extent, this could be understood as an instance of compensatory justice (see above). In one form or another, however, it would amount to granting women preferential treatment in biomedical research. Going beyond the distributive model, in which women must be represented fairly in relation to their health risk in clinical studies likely to benefit the subject population, this conception of justice holds that those who are currently oppressed in society should have a privileged place in studies that are likely to be of specific benefit to members of the group investigated.

A final model of justice goes beyond considerations of distribution and oppression to address questions of power and influence over the process of setting the research agenda. Although it may seem that the notions of "benefit" and "burden" can be objectively defined, different groups may construe the burdens of being a research participant in a variety of ways. Moreover, the health priorities of a study population may not be the same as the priorities of those who set the research agenda.

Being part of the process that establishes a research agenda can be construed as a requirement of procedural justice. This point is illustrated by the history of acquired immune deficiency syndrome (AIDS) research. Much of the initial research on AIDS understandably focused on gay and bisexual men, because they were the first population identified as having the disease in sizable numbers. This focus is not only gender-specific. Even after male intravenous drug users were known to be afflicted with AIDS, only rarely were they recruited as research subjects. When research interest first focused on women with HIV infection, the concern was largely for their role as "vectors" rather than as patients: "the original interest in HIV-infected women centered on their relation to pediatric AIDS through perinatal transmission. A search of the medical literature yields only a handful of papers focusing on the consequences of the infection in nonpregnant women" (Mitchell et al., 1992; see also C. Levine, 1990; Faden et al., in press).

This picture of enrollment in AIDS research reveals equal class and gender bias. Because the primary population initially infected was gay men, it is understandable that a much larger proportion of men than women were subjects. At some point, however, the failure to focus on the health interests of women affected by the epidemic is considered by many to have become inappropriate. Most of the women who have acquired HIV disease from intravenous drug use or from having sexual relations with IV drug users are also poor and members of diverse racial and ethnic groups; they have been inadequately represented in AIDS research not only as women, but also (along with male IV drug users) as poor members of racial and ethnic groups.

For the nation's research agenda to be just, it must ensure that medical research promotes the health and well-being of both men and women. Where it is established that women or other groups have not received a fair allocation of research attention or resources, justice may require that the research agenda provide preferential treatment in these areas. To set a just research agenda for the nation may thus require more than a reordering of priorities. It may also require substantial changes in the way funding priorities are established, to ensure that the objectives of a research program coincide with the health benefits sought by specific communities of potential research participants. Changes also may be required in the way funds are allocated generally and for women's health issues specifically, as well as some administrative restructuring of funding agencies. We will have more to say about how to implement these principles of justice in Chapter 8.

## LIMITS TO THE REQUIREMENTS OF JUSTICE

There is an important limit to the requirements of justice with respect to gender in the conduct of clinical studies. If it is true that women or members of poorer groups or some racial and ethnic groups have not been included in research in appropriate numbers, do the demands of justice now impose on them an *obligation* to serve as subjects? Does redressing past imbalances or ensuring justice in the future require that groups that have been *excluded* must now be *recruited?*

The answer to these questions marks the boundary between ethical and unethical recruitment. The requirements of distributive justice demand that recruitment efforts fulfill the criteria outlined in this chapter, but the ethical requirement of *voluntariness of participation* in research sets limits on what might actually be achievable. The obligations of justice for inclusion of different groups in research are thus imposed on the scientific community and its sponsors, not on the subject populations to be enrolled.

Researchers may now stand to gain or lose directly in accordance with their success in recruiting a diverse study sample. The gain, if in compliance with inclusiveness, may be a higher priority for funding or the ability to receive continuation funds. The penalty for noncompliance may be losing research funds. This situation will produce strong incentives to researchers to enroll a diverse study sample.

The participants themselves, however, may not benefit from the research. Even in studies that promise enhanced benefits from an investigational drug, a control group receiving a placebo or the standard treatment will not receive the enhanced benefits by serving as research subjects. It is the investigator's responsibility to see that the needs and rights of potential participants are balanced against the need to have them in the study. To guard against potential exploitation and manipulation in the recruitment of particularly "desirable" subjects, every effort must be made to balance the pressure to encourage the inclusion of women—and particularly women from diverse racial and ethnic groups and the poor—with the equally appropriate pressure to heighten investigators' awareness of the importance of soliciting valid, voluntary consents.

The requirement of valid consent does not preclude appropriate compensation to participants for time lost from work, costs of travel to the research site, baby-sitting expenses, or any other out-of-pocket costs incurred by research subjects. If justice requires recruitment of research subjects from all social, economic, and ethnic groups, it also requires that volunteers be compensated for any financial losses they incur from serving as subjects. At the same time, incentives for participation should not be so great as to constitute an undue inducement to participate. If investigators offer monetary or other incentives to poor people that unduly influence them to enroll, what is gained by meeting the requirement of distributive justice is lost by diminishing the voluntariness of participation (see Chapter 5).

## STATEMENT OF GUIDING PRINCIPLES

Based on the foregoing examination, the committee recommends three general principles of justice with regard to issues of inclusion of both genders in the conduct of clinical research:

1.  The scientific community and the institutions that support it must ensure that scientific advances in medicine and public health fairly benefit all people, regardless of gender, race, ethnicity, or age. Therefore, the national research agenda must ensure that medical research promotes the health and well-being of both women and men.

2.  Where it is established that specific health interests of women, men, or other groups have not received a fair allocation of research attention or resources, justice may require a policy of preferential treatment

toward these specific areas in order to remedy a past injustice and to avoid perpetuating that injustice.

3.   Volunteers for clinical studies should be offered the opportunity to participate without regard to gender, race, ethnicity, or age. Women and men should be enrolled as participants in clinical studies in a manner that ensures that research yields scientifically generalizable results applicable to both genders.

These principles guide the committee's deliberations in the following chapters, which examine the challenges to applying these principles, and achieving equity in clinical studies, that arise from four specific areas: scientific considerations (Chapter 4); social and ethical considerations (Chapter 5); legal considerations (Chapter 6); and issues surrounding risks to reproduction and offspring (Chapter 7).

## REFERENCES

DeBruin, D.A. 1994. Justice and the inclusion of women in clinical studies: A conceptual framework. In: Women and Health Research: Ethical and Legal Issues of Including Women in Clinical Studies, Volume 2, A. Mastroianni, R. Faden, and D. Federman, eds. Washington, D.C.: National Academy Press.

Faden, R., Kass, N., and McGraw, D. In press. Women as vessels and vectors: Lessons from the HIV epidemic. In: Feminism and Bioethics: Beyond Reproduction, S. Wolf, ed. New York: Oxford University Press.

Levine, C. 1990. Women and HIV/AIDS research: The barriers to equity. *Evaluation Review* 14(5):447-463.

Mitchell, J.L., et al. 1992. HIV and Women: Current controversies and clinical relevance, *Journal of Women's Health* 1(1):35-39.

National Commission for the Protection of Human Subjects of Biomedical and Behavioral Research. 1978. The Belmont Report: Ethical Principles and Guidelines for the Protection of Human Subjects of Research. Washington, D.C.: Government Printing Office.

Special Programme of Research, Development and Research Training in Human Reproduction and International Women's Health Coalition. 1991. Creating Common Ground: Women's Perspectives on the Selection and Introduction of Fertility Regulation Technologies. Geneva: World Health Organization.

Sherwin, S. 1994. Women in Clinical Studies: A feminist view. In: Women and Health Research: The Ethical and Legal Issues of Including Women in Clinical Studies, Volume 2, A. Mastroianni, R. Faden, and D. Federman, eds. Washington, D.C.: National Academy Press.

Young, I.M. 1990. Justice and the Politics of Difference. Princeton, N.J.: Princeton University Press.

# 4

# Scientific Considerations

Implicit in the guiding principles developed in Chapter 3 is the assumption that there *are* meaningful differences between the sexes, and that—at least in some instances—the results of male-only studies cannot be reliably or safely generalized to women. This chapter examines the scientific evidence for that assumption and its implications for the design of clinical studies. Both of these issues have consequences for a policy of inclusion, as mandated by the NIH Revitalization Act of 1993.

There is a general belief among clinical researchers that, in most situations, women and men will *not* differ significantly in their response to treatment. The evidence to support this belief is not easily assembled, however, and there are countervailing concerns that gender differences have been insufficiently studied. Some of the known gender differences in response to treatments are related to physiological differences between the genders. Important examples include hormonal differences, particularly the variation in drug response by women during different stages of the menstrual cycle, and pharmacokinetic effects such as differential rates of drug absorption and excretion. Other differences are psychosocial in origin or are mediated by tendencies of men and women to act differently with respect to health care. In cases where there is substantial evidence of a qualitative or large quantitative difference in response by gender, the weight of evidence supports a policy of including both genders in sufficient number to permit subgroup analyses, except in studies involving conditions or treatments that affect only one gender.

These true gender differences (and differences associated with gender, e.g., weight) have implications for the design of clinical trials, the subset of clinical studies that provides the most rigorous and reliable test of the effectiveness and safety of new drugs and treatments. For example, greater heterogeneity among research subjects may permit the investigator to spot trends that might otherwise be missed, even if the numbers are too small for statistically reliable subgroup analysis. At the same time, greater homogeneity among research subjects reduces unexplained variance.

## EVIDENCE OF GENDER DIFFERENCES

This report, originating as it does from concerns about insufficient attention being directed toward identifying and understanding gender differences, of necessity highlights diseases and treatments that can differ by gender in a variety of ways. Differences can arise from a range of factors, both biological (e.g., the effect of endogenous or exogenous hormones or gender-related differences in body mass, etc.) and psychosocial (e.g., gender-related differences in behaviors such as smoking or substance abuse). The question that must be addressed is to what extent are gender differences per se clinically meaningful in the treatment of conditions involving both genders?

Most clinical researchers and clinicians would argue that women and men do not respond significantly differently to the presence of disease or the effect of treatment. Even for diseases where women and men differ significantly in the likely time of onset (such as heart disease), they will usually respond in much the same way to treatment and experience a similar evolution of the disease. The underlying reasons for this belief are rooted in several observations regarding health problems relevant to both men and women: for the majority of drug treatments, efficacy and safety do not depend on such factors as body mass, adipose tissue, hormones, or other factors associated with gender. Treatments by surgical procedure for diseases associated with both genders seldom differ because the patient is a woman instead of a man; and to the extent that women may be treated differently, it is because of factors associated with gender but not specific to gender, such as bone mass or organ size. Finally, a long history of nonhuman research—ranging from work with bacteria to research with mammals—supports the conclusion that subgroup differences are rare. Most treatments and disease processes are thus thought to be insensitive to gender per se. Nevertheless, the evidentiary base for quantifying these claims in humans is weak because the relevant data have not been organized into an accessible format and the claim is seldom questioned.

At the same time, concern is mounting among both scientific observers and lay representatives that researchers and clinicians may be too quick to *assume* there are no differences between women and men, rather than *test* for gender-related effects. Much of the controversy surrounding the issue of women's participation in clinical studies has centered on differential responses to drugs between men and women. Significant gender differences in drug response have not been detected in the majority of cases, but where they are detected they can be important. Therefore, it becomes important for clinical investigators to ascertain under what conditions such gender differences are likely to occur and to design clinical studies accordingly. The following sections summarize some of the literature on documented gender differences, primarily with respect to differences in drug response.

## Body Size, Composition, and Metabolism

Men and women differ in body size, body composition, and metabolism (Table 4-1). On average, women are smaller than men in weight, height, and surface area (Silvaggio and Mattison, 1993). This may affect drug dosing, which may be more appropriately based on body weight (or surface area) than on a fixed dose. It is of interest that most adult dosing is done on a fixed dose, not based on weight or surface area.

For example, if a drug is administered on the basis of body weight (say 10 mg/kg), then a typical adult male will receive a dose of 700 mg and a typical adult female 570 mg. If the same drug is given on the basis of surface area (say, 380 mg/m), then the average adult male will receive a dose of 703 mg and the average female 608 mg. If weight or surface area are not taken into consideration, however, and men and women are given the same dose (700 mg, for example), then the average male will get a dose of 10.0 mg/kg and the average female 12.2 mg/kg. If the drug has minimal toxicity or a wide therapeutic index, these differences in dosage may be of little consequence. If the therapeutic index is narrow, however, or the toxicity severe, these differences may be of critical importance.

Compared with men, women also have a lower ratio of lean body mass to adipose (fatty) tissue (Yonkers et al., 1992). This difference in body composition may affect drug disposition—for example, the water content and metabolism of adipose tissue differs from that in muscle tissue (Silvaggio and Mattison, 1993). Lipid-soluble drugs such as the benzodiazepines would be expected to have a greater volume of distribution in women (on the basis of body weight or surface area), which would affect the appropriate therapeutic dose.

For all ages after sexual maturation, metabolism (as measured by basal metabolic rates) is higher in men. Drug metabolism differences by gender have been poorly studied. A few drugs, however, demonstrate gender differences in metabolism, including nicotine, acetylsalicylic acid (aspirin), and heparin (an anticoagulant) (Silvaggio and Mattison, 1993).

TABLE 4-1 Representative Values of Weight, Height, Surface Area, and Caloric Intake for Adult Males and Females

| Sex | Weight (kg) | Height (cm) | Surface Area (m$^2$) | Caloric Intake | Kilocalories/ Kilogram[a] | Kilocalories/ Meter |
|---|---|---|---|---|---|---|
| Male | 70.0 | 178 | 1.85 | 3,000 | 43 | 1,620 |
| Female | 57.0 | 163 | 1.60 | 2,300 | 40 | 1,440 |

[a]Kilocalories per kilogram are given to indicate the significant differences in metabolic rate when calculated on the basis of body weight.

SOURCE: NRC, 1993.

TABLE 4-2  Concentrations of Steroids/Hormones in
Males and Females

| Item by Gender | Concentration |
|---|---|
| Estrogen (urinary) | |
|   Males | 5-40  n mole/24 h |
|   Females | |
|     <10 years | 0.5 |
|     follicular | 20-150 |
|     mid-cycle | 60-300 |
|     luteal phase | 45-290 |
|     post-menopausal | 10-55 |
| Progesterone (plasma) | |
|   Males | <5 n mole/L |
|   Females | 15-77 n mole/L |
| Prolactin (plasma) | |
|   Males | <450 U/L |
|   Females | <600 U/L |
| Testosterone | |
|   Males | 14-42 n mole/L |
|   Females | 1-2.1 |

SOURCE: Wetherall et al., 1988.

Another obvious difference between men and women is the presence of
hormones such as estrogen, progesterone, prolactin, and testosterone (Table
4-2). These hormonal differences are important for establishing and maintaining a range of gender-dependent physiological characteristics. They may
also modify the pharmacokinetics and pharmacodynamics of selected drugs.

Gender differences may also be found in other commonly measured
laboratory tests such as serum iron, uric acid, creatinine phosphokinase, and
gamma glutamyl transpeptidase, all of which are important in distinguishing
the normal from the abnormal in selected disease states (Table 4-3).

TABLE 4-3  Concentrations ($\mu$ mole/liter) of Commonly
Measured Tests in Males and Females

| Group | Serum Iron | Uric Acid | Creatine Phospho-kinase | Gamma Glutamyl Transpeptidase |
|---|---|---|---|---|
| Males | 14-31 | 210-480 | 25-195 | 11-51 |
| Females | 11-30 | 150-390 | 25-170 | 7-33 |

SOURCE: Wetherall et al., 1988

## Gender and Aging

Men and women over the age of 65 currently make up 13 percent of the total population in this country, a percentage that is expected to grow significantly in the coming decades (Olshansky et al., 1993). Because women live longer than men by an average of 7 years, they presently constitute a majority (59 percent) of those over 65 and nearly 75 percent of those over the age of 85. While many of the medically relevant differences that exist between younger men and women persist into older age, men and women over 65 also experience gender-associated health problems that are unique to their age group.

Frequently associated with advanced age, for instance, is the increased use of medications. Men and women over the age of 65 consume 30 percent of all prescription drugs sold in the United States (NIA, 1992). Of this amount, women consume 20 percent more drugs than men (National Medical Expenditure Survey, 1987). For women over 65, this translates into an average consumption of 5.7 prescriptions a year, not including the average consumption of 3.2 over-the-counter drugs a year by this group (National Center for Health Statistics, 1985). One-quarter of women over 65 consume as many as 21 different medications in a year; one-fifth of men over 65 consume this many medications in a year (National Medical Expenditure Survey, 1987).

Women over 65 suffer more adverse events related to medication than do men in the same age group, although these events are more likely to result in death for males. For both genders, cardiac, antihypertensive, and nonsteroidal anti-inflammatory agents are the most common causes of these events (Tanner et al., 1989). Adverse events may also occur in both sexes with the use of water-soluble drugs such as lithium. Although older men and women both experience decreases in lean body mass and increases in fat tissue as a fraction of body weight, these changes may be more pronounced in women, who tend to have more body fat than males in youth and middle age. As a result, drugs such as lithium may have a more immediate toxic effect in older women (Everitt and Avorn, 1986). In addition, lipophilic drugs such as phenothiazines and many benzodiazepines may have a more prolonged effect in older women.

Men and women over 65 also differ with respect to the diseases and conditions that commonly affect them. For example, older women are affected by rheumatoid arthritis three times more frequently than men, while men over 65 are affected by gout in significantly greater numbers (NIA, 1992). Osteoporosis is far more common in women than men, affecting slightly over 73 percent of women aged 65-69 and 89 percent of women over age 75 (NIH, 1992). Women develop osteoporosis with advanced age as a result of decreased hormone levels, too little calcium in the diet, inactivity, and perhaps heredity; men appear to be protected from the disease by denser bone structure and other factors (NIA, 1992). In addition to osteoporosis, women over 65 experience other chronic conditions with greater frequency than men in the same age group, including digestive disorders and thyroid diseases.

Mental health problems also afflict older women to a greater extent than older men. Women over 65 experience depression four times as often as men; anxiety disorders, sleep disorders, mania, and late-onset psychosis also occur more frequently in older women (NIH, 1992). Neurodegenerative diseases such as Alzheimer's disease and certain movement disorders also affect women disproportionately, although it is unclear whether this reflects brain differences or simply differences in survival. Evidence for the latter hypothesis is strong: the majority of Alzheimer's disease patients are over the age of 80, an age when women outnumber men nearly two to one (NIH Advisory Committee on Women's Health Issues, 1988).

Just as sources of morbidity differ between men and women over 65, so too do causes of mortality. Older men die from heart disease and malignant neoplasms more frequently than do older women, who die more often from cerebrovascular disease (National Center for Health Statistics, 1993). Nevertheless, these three diseases remain the top killers of all persons over the age of 65.

## Behavioral and Psychosocial Differences

Men and women also differ in a number of psychosocial variables that can affect disease risk, treatment, or prevention. These variables mainly pertain to gender roles and lifestyle (Rodin and Ickovics, 1990). There are stresses associated with the multiple roles women typically assume in taking on the responsibilities of balancing work and family, but the evidence of negative effects from this source of stress on women's health is inconclusive (Horton, 1992). Women also are more likely to experience domestic violence leading to physical and psychological injuries (Rodin and Ickovics, 1990). Twice as many women as men experience major depression, and a number of psychosocial factors have been found to be risk factors for depression in women, including imbalances in perceived control over one's life, social support, and sense of accomplishment and independence (McGrath et al., 1990; Horton, 1992).

Gender differences in lifestyle may also affect health. Women tend to get less regular exercise than men, and a sedentary lifestyle has been linked to cardiovascular disease in men (National Women's Health Resource Center, 1990). More men than women drink alcohol and smoke tobacco, but increased consumption of both substances by women over the past few decades poses serious risks to women's health. Because cigarette smoking is an important risk factor for numerous diseases—including heart disease, lung cancer, and chronic obstructive pulmonary disease—the rise in smoking among adolescent and young women is of special concern. There is increasing evidence that even moderate use of alcohol increases the risk for breast cancer in women by 50 percent (Rodin and Ickovics, 1990).

Cultural emphasis on thinness and beauty in women translate into a higher prevalence of eating disorders, such as anorexia nervosa and bulimia (Horton, 1992) and high use of over-the-counter diet pills (women constitute 90 percent of users) (Rodin and Ickovics, 1990). The poor nutrition in childhood and adolescence that results from such dieting creates a greater risk for osteoporosis in later life. The desire for thinness has also been implicated in women smokers' reluctance to quit, because the average quitter gains about five pounds (Horton, 1992). The pressure to be thin may also affect women's compliance with drug regimens when the side effects include weight gain (National Women's Health Resource Center, 1990).

## Endogenous Hormones

Not all gender differences are merely a matter of degree; some are specific to one gender. From menarche to menopause, women undergo cyclical physiological changes, with a duration of approximately 28 days, known as the menstrual cycle. The menses are characterized by low levels of the hormones estrogen and progesterone. During the follicular phase, the level of estrogen rises and the endometrium thickens to enable a fertilized ovum to implant if conception occurs during that cycle. During the luteal phase, following ovulation, the level of estrogen declines and the level of progesterone rises. If fertilization and implantation do not occur, the level of progesterone declines and the menses begin a new cycle.

Endogenous hormonal changes in menstruating women can affect drug disposition, but few studies have examined the impact of changing hormonal concentrations on drug metabolism across the different phases of the menstrual cycle (GAO, 1992; NRC, 1993). One recent report noted the importance of varying the dose of an antidepressant over the menstrual cycle to achieve optimal benefit and minimal side effects (Jensvold et al., 1992). Thus, although rarely studied, there is some evidence that while constant drug dosing may be appropriate for males, females may benefit from variable dosing tailored to their menstrual cycles.

Endogenous hormones may also affect the success of some types of surgical treatments. For example, recent studies suggest a potential link between the timing (within the menstrual cycle) of surgery for breast cancer and the rate of recurrence and survival (NRC, 1993). Multivariate analyses, controlling for such variables as tumor size and number of lymph nodes involved, suggest that surgery during the early luteal phase of the cycle enhances survival, although the exact reason is undetermined.

### Pregnancy and Lactation

Numerous physiological changes occur during pregnancy, and some of these changes persist during lactation. Beyond changing the size, shape, and center of gravity in the body, changes occur in the pulmonary, cardiovascular, renal, gastrointestinal, and hepatic systems. These changes can alter the body's disposition of drugs, including absorption, distribution, metabolism, and elimination (Hytten and Leitch, 1971; Hytten and Chamberlain 1980; Mattison and Jelovsek, 1991; Mattison et al., 1992; Mattison 1986, 1990). Table 4-4 lists some of these physiological changes and their pharmacokinetic effects.

Some of the changes that occur during pregnancy, such as increased plasma volume, body weight, and body fat, can decrease the concentration

TABLE 4-4  Changes During Pregnancy that May Alter Pharmacokinetics

| Pharmacokinetic Parameter | Change | Pharmacokinetic Impact |
|---|---|---|
| Absorption | | |
|     Gastric emptying time | Increased | Increased absorption and/or metabolism |
|     Intestinal motility | Decreased | Increased absorption |
|     Pulmonary function | Increased | Increased absorption and/or elimination |
|     Cardiac output | Increased | Increased distribution rate |
|     Blood flow to the skin | Increased | Increased transdermal absorption |
| Distribution | | |
|     Plasma volume | Increased | Increased volume of distribution |
|     Total body water | Increased | Increased volume of distribution |
|     Plasma proteins | Decreased | Decreased volume of distribution, decreased binding capacity |
|     Body fat | Increased | Increased volume of distribution, increased reservoir for lipid-soluble xenobiotics |
| Metabolism | | |
|     Hepatic metabolism | +/- | +/- Metabolic alteration and elimination |
|     Extra-hepatic metabolism | +/- | +/- Metabolic alteration and elimination |
|     Plasma proteins | Decreased | Increased metabolic alteration and elimination |
| Excretion | | |
|     Renal blood flow | Increased | Increased renal elimination |
|     Glomerular filtration rate | Increased | Increased renal elimination |
|     Pulmonary function | Increased | Increased pulmonary elimination |
|     Plasma proteins | Decreased | +/- Elimination |

SOURCE: Modified from Mattison, 1986.

of a drug in the body, thereby decreasing its therapeutic effect. Pregnant women with epilepsy, for example, typically require higher doses of phenytoin (by 50 percent or more) to avoid seizures than nonpregnant women. Other changes, such as decreased intestinal motility and decreased gastric emptying time, can cause a drug to be absorbed in greater amounts than when a woman is not pregnant. These circumstances may warrant decreasing dosage of some drugs during pregnancy. In addition to changing maternal drug disposition, both the placenta and fetus can contribute to modified drug disposition (Gillette, 1977; Pelkonen, 1980). These effects, however, are thought to be small compared with maternal effects on the drug.

It may be ideal for women to avoid medication altogether while pregnant, but this can be difficult (see also Chapter 7). A wide array of maternal, fetal, and pregnancy-associated conditions can require treatment during pregnancy, and as many as 75 percent of pregnant women use prescription or over-the-counter drugs—hence the importance of understanding the pharmacokinetic changes that occur during pregnancy.

Many of the physiological changes that occur with pregnancy persist for some time after childbirth, so their impact on a nursing infant must also be considered in drug dosing. Factors that determine the concentration of drugs in breast milk include dosing interval, frequency of breastfeeding, and lipid solubility. Because breast milk is rich in lipids (3 to 5 percent by volume), lipid-soluble drugs are preferentially found in breast milk. Although most drugs taken by the mother are found in breast milk, the dose to the infant is typically small.

### Exogenous Hormones

### Hormonal Contraceptives

Data from a 1988 survey indicate that 31 percent of U.S. women between the ages of 15 and 44 use oral contraceptives (OCs) (Mosher, 1990). Most OCs are pills that contain synthetic hormones, usually estrogen and progestin, although some OCs contain only a progestin compound. In addition to being highly effective in preventing pregnancy, OCs also reduce the risk of ovarian and endometrial cancer. Two other long-acting hormonal contraceptives that contain only progestins have recently become available— Norplant® and DepoProvera®—and close to a million U.S. women are now using these methods.

Despite their many health benefits, OCs also have adverse effects. For example, OCs have been found to increase the risk of coronary heart disease, particularly acute myocardial infarction, a risk that is compounded in smokers. Most of the studies linking OCs to heart disease, however, are based on women who took pills containing much higher doses of estrogen and progestin than are contained in pills used today. More research is needed to assess the effects of lower-dose OCs on the risk of cardiovascular disease in smokers and nonsmokers (National Women's Health Resource Center, 1990).

Oral contraceptives can also influence the pharmacokinetics and pharmacodynamics of other drugs. For example, the ethinyl estradiol component of OCs is responsible for reducing hepatic metabolism of many drugs, thereby increasing plasma concentrations (e.g., prednisolone, antipyrine, imipramine, diazepam, chlordiazepoxide, phenytoin, caffeine, and cyclosporine) (Teichmann, 1990; NRC, 1993). For other drugs, OCs can induce drug metabolism, thus lowering plasma concentrations (as with acetaminophen, morphine, lorazepam, and oxazepam) (NRC, 1993). Drug interactions can also reduce the efficacy of OCs themselves; anticonvulsants in particular are known to reduce OC concentrations and effectiveness.

### Menopause and Hormone Replacement

Menopause, the time in a woman's life when the production of estrogen declines and menstruation ceases, usually occurs sometime between the mid-forties and early fifties. Many signs and symptoms accompany the onset of menopause, including hot flashes, irritability, and sleep disturbances (Bush, 1992). Estrogen replacement therapy has been recommended to reduce or eliminate these unpleasant symptoms, as well as to prevent the development of osteoporosis by reducing bone loss in the immediate postmenopausal period (Bush, 1992).

Observational studies indicate that estrogen, alone or in combination with progestin, is associated with a 50 percent reduction in the risk of cardiovascular disease. Oral (as opposed to transdermal) estrogens alter plasma lipoproteins, raising levels of high-density lipoprotein cholesterol ("good" cholesterol) and lowering levels of low-density lipoprotein cholesterol (Matthews et al., 1989; Stampfer et al., 1991; NIH Consensus Development Panel on Triglyceride, High Density Lipoprotein, and Coronary Heart Disease, 1993). Combination hormonal therapy (estrogen and progestin together) may offer an advantage over estrogen alone in altering cardiovascular risk factors (Nabulsi et al., 1993). Studies of the effect of postmenopausal hormone use on the risk of stroke have produced conflicting results, some showing no effect, others showing a benefit, and still others showing an increased risk (Stampfer et al., 1991; Finucane et al., 1993).

There are other risks associated with estrogen or combined hormonal therapies. An increased risk of endometrial cancer has been associated with estrogen use, although this risk diminishes with the addition of a progestin (Bush, 1992). Whether or not hormone replacement increased the risk of breast cancer is unresolved (Horton, 1992). Recent data suggest that the combination hormone therapy may increase the risk of breast cancer (Bush, 1992).

## METHODOLOGICAL IMPLICATIONS

All of these gender differences are relevant to the design of clinical drug trials. Differences in size, fat ratios, and metabolic rates are associated with differences in drug concentration, metabolism, and response. Psychosocial differences are associated with differences in risk factors and, more important, in adherence to experimental protocols. These differences can change over time, both in the short term (during the menstrual cycle) and the long term (with pregnancy, lactation, and aging). The relevance of these factors and their potential impacts on study design, particularly in issues of inclusion or exclusion of subjects, merit a closer look.

### Clinical Studies

A *study* for purposes of this discussion is any experimental or nonexperimental investigation or analysis of a question, process, or phenomenon. In a broad sense, the term is used to refer to any one of a variety of activities involving the collection, analysis, or interpretation of data. Strictly defined, the adjective *clinical* means relating to a clinic or sickbed or to care rendered in a clinic or at the bedside of the sick. More broadly, the term simply serves to identify that which has or is thought to have some medical relevance to the treatment, prevention, or amelioration of disease.

Hence, a *clinical study* in this context refers to any investigation or analysis of a question, process, or phenomenon that has, or is presumed to have, some immediate or future clinical relevance. The class of studies included in this general category include all of those performed on human beings for the general purpose of learning more about processes of health, disease, and disability and for the specific purpose of developing and testing treatments and procedures used for health maintenance and for treatment of disease. Also included are studies performed without any contact with people, instead using data generated from the observation or treatment of people (e.g., studies based on medical records).

For the remainder of this chapter, however, we focus on *clinical trials*, and particularly treatment trials, as an important subset of clinical studies. There are two related reasons for this focus: (1) the most vexing ethical and legal issues attend clinical studies of the therapeutic efficacy of treatment interventions and (2) clinical trials are considered to be the most rigorous test of therapeutic efficacy of drugs or other clinical interventions. Consequently, concerns about the potential for compromising the scientific merit of clinical research through implementation of changes in NIH policy regarding inclusion of women will have their greatest relevance for this set of designs. We recognize that many of the scientific considerations reviewed here also apply to other designs and clinical studies; some, however, are particularly cogent for clinical trials of treatment interventions.

## Clinical Trials

In the broadest usage, a *clinical trial* is an experiment designed to assess the safety and efficacy of one treatment relative to another in comparable groups of human beings treated according to a given protocol and observed for change in an outcome measure or for occurrence of some event. In the most restrictive view, the modifier *clinical* should be reserved for the subset of trials that is done in a clinical setting and based on outcome measures with obvious clinical implications. As used in this report, the term is assigned to the subset of trials characterized as being *controlled* (i.e., having two or more comparable treatment groups concurrently enrolled and treated). There is no stipulation of how comparability is to be achieved; *randomized* trials represent a subset of clinical trials and the larger set of trials in general.

*Crossover trials* involve designs in which participants receive two or more of the study treatments in some designated order. *Parallel trials* are characterized by treatment structures lacking such crossing: persons enrolled are assigned to receive only one of the study treatments. The typical crossover trial involves relatively short follow-up periods and usually has some laboratory test or measure as the outcome of interest; it may or may not involve people with clinical disease.

It is also useful to distinguish between two general classes of sample size designs—*sequential* and *fixed*. Trials of the former type are carried out without a predetermined sample size requirement: the number of people enrolled or the time it is allowed to run are determined by the differences observed during the trial. Fixed sample size designs enroll a predetermined number of participants, typically dictated by a sample size calculation or other considerations (e.g., the cost or availability of patients). More generally, any nonsequential sample size design, even if the sample size is not fixed or determined before the start of the trial, is considered to be a fixed sample size design. The discussion that follows focuses on fixed sample size designs.

## External and Internal Validity

Some of the methodological concerns raised about gender equity in clinical trials (and clinical studies more generally) are rooted in concerns about *external validity;* that is, the ability to generalize the findings obtained from a sample to a broader population. These arguments are reflected, implicitly or explicitly, in other chapters, for example in the concerns that clinicians and patients may be confused about whether a treatment that has been tested only on men is also effective—and safe—for women with the same disease.

These concerns about generalizability have merit, but the external validity of clinical trials, as a methodological issue, is an oxymoron. External validity per se derives from drawing a representative sample of the population of interest. Other types of clinical studies that use survey techniques to sample randomly (say, from all Medicare patients hospitalized for gall bladder surgery) might claim to have external validity for describing the entire population (i.e., all Medicare patients with hospitalization for gall bladder surgery, and perhaps non-Medicare patients as well). Clinical trials, however, do not take a random sample from a representative population. Instead, they screen volunteers to see if they meet the selection criteria (see below) and then randomize the participants into treatment or nontreatment subgroups. This kind of design focuses instead on achieving *internal validity*—that is, how consistently and how well the treatment works. In this sense clinical trials, as a design, cannot truly speak to external validity issues; nevertheless, they can speak to gender differences in treatment effect, and in that sense can contribute to the knowledge and understanding of whether women and men differ in their responses to treatment.

### Homogeneity Versus Heterogeneity

In order to assess the effect of treatments, clinical investigators try to reduce or eliminate sources of variance that are under their control, although they cannot achieve the same degree of control as the laboratory scientist. Hence, they construct criteria for the selection of subjects, criteria that are intended to reduce variance by recruiting the most homogeneous sample possible. From the narrow perspective of a single trial, the more homogeneous the population, the better. From this perspective, heterogeneity holds no intrinsic value and is simply the end result of not having been able to achieve the desired degree of homogeneity because of the costs involved (measured by effort or by dollars) or because of other limitations or constraints.

The smaller the anticipated sample size of the trial, the more important it is to recruit a homogeneous sample with regard to factors known to affect treatment. There are two reasons for this:

1. Variations in the population enrolled in a small trial can have greater effect on the results than in a large trial. Randomization is more likely to do its "job" in a large trial than in a small one: a "bad break" in the randomiza-

tion process in relation to patient characteristics is more likely to be "confounding" in a small trial than in a large one.

2.   The ability to adjust for differences in the composition of the study groups (e.g., through regression techniques) is limited if not completely precluded in a small trial, whereas it is the method of choice for adjustment in the large trial.

## Exclusions from Trials

As a general rule, the list of exclusions should be as short as possible, and each exclusion should be justified on medical or scientific grounds. The list should be pared by an active process of review and challenge prior to the start of the trial, and the list should be periodically reviewed during the trial for possible further trimming. Typical reasons for excluding patients from clinical trials include any or all of the following:

*   *Disease stage* (the disease is too advanced or not advanced enough for the treatment being studied; prognosis inconsistent with treatment).
*   *Clinical contraindications* (e.g., allergy to one of the study drugs).
*   *Regulatory or ethical restrictions* (study drug not approved for use in children; subject is incapable of giving valid informed consent to participation, for example).
*   *Compliance considerations* (e.g., history of illegal intravenous drug use in a drug trial requiring an indwelling line for drug infusion).
*   *Variance control* (including age restrictions because of anticipated differences in response to treatment by age group).

In every instance, exclusions should be based on strong supporting data in published documents. The first four reasons, assuming that they are based on well-reasoned evidence, can all be defended as being important for the validity of the study. The last general reason for exclusion, variance control, is where gender restrictions have been most often imposed (to achieve homogeneity) without actual evidence to suspect gender differences. Within broad limits, selection criteria related to the disease under scrutiny are sufficient to ensure scientifically based homogeneity; the addition of demographic variables adds little, particularly in treatment trials.

In general, there are two justifications for excluding subjects on the basis of demographic characteristics such as gender, race, ethnicity, or age: (1) when these demographic statuses serve as surrogates for some other risk factor (as would be needed in a risk-concentration design) or (2) when the disease or condition being treated is concentrated in a particular subgroup (e.g., sickle cell anemia in African Americans or breast cancer in women). The mere fact that the number of any demographic subgroup enrolled in a study would be too small to permit statistically valid subgroup analyses (such as women in a study of MIs) does not constitute a valid scientific reason for their exclusion. The arguments that the ability to detect the main effect because of the added variance arising from inclusion of both genders are generally without scientific validity; in most cases, the study group can be "homogenized" by carrying out statistical analyses taking gender and other factors into account.

*Age-based exclusions*   These issues can be illustrated by examining the age- and gender-based rationales for exclusions from several commonly cited male-only trials of conditions and treatments applicable to both men and women. In the Coronary Drug Project, for example, the rationale for the *lower* age limit of 35 had to do with the epidemiology of heart disease (that is, women and men alike experience relatively few MIs before that age) and the medical postulate that MIs occurring before 35 may be different from those occurring later in life (CDPRG, 1973). In the Multiple Risk Factor Intervention Trial (MRFIT), the rationale for the lower age limit of 35 was based on compliance-related considerations (MRFIT Group, 1977). Because the treatments involved sustained lifestyle changes, the study excluded the portion of the population (under 35) believed to be problematic in making and sustaining dietary changes in cholesterol intake.

The rationale for *upper* age limits in adult populations is different. Often they are imposed in prevention trials to ensure sufficient remaining lifetime to allow the treatment to have an effect or to concentrate on the portion of the population believed able to benefit from the treatment. Such exclusions, however, should not be imposed without reference to the duration considered necessary, on average, to accrue treatment benefits, and they should not be used without an understanding of conditional life expectancies. Generally, most people well enough to walk into a clinic and enroll in a secondary prevention trial have several years of remaining life, regardless of their age. In 1989, for example, the conditional life expectancy at age 70 was 12.1 years for a white male, 11.0 for a black male, 15.3 for a white female, and 13.9 for a black female; the corresponding figures at age 85 were 5.3 for a white male, 6.5 for a white female, 5.6 for a black male, and 6.7 for a black female (U.S. Bureau of the Census, 1992).

*Gender-based exclusions*   More germane to this report are the rationales underlying the exclusion of women from two large preventive clinical trials: the Physicians' Health Study and MRFIT. The primary reason for excluding women from the Physicians' Health Study was the gender mix of the physician cohort approached for study (approximately 90 percent male); the number of women in the cohort was not large enough for a gender-by-treatment interaction analysis. The investigators' reservations regarding the ability to perform such an analysis were sound, but the enrollment of a specified subgroup does not obligate them to perform interaction analysis for that subgroup, nor does the analysis need to be definitive if performed. If nothing else, the sign and size of any difference observed for women would have provided some general indication of whether the result obtained in men is consistent with that observed in, and thus generalizable to, women.

Another possible argument for excluding women from clinical trials is that of efficiency: is the increase in information gained proportionate to the increased costs of including women? If including women would have resulted in a 10 percent increase in person-years of follow-up information, for example, then to justify excluding them it would have been necessary to show that adding women would have increased costs by more than 10 percent. In the case of the Physicians' Health Study, including women would probably have added valuable follow-up information without adding disproportionate costs. Most of its costs had to do with its coordinating center and other central functions; the cost for screening, treatment, and follow-up of each participant were relatively low.

The basis for the gender exclusion in MRFIT is more compelling on both scientific and practical grounds. Screening costs were higher than those of the Physicians' Health Study because it was necessary to find people with a defined risk profile based on smoking behavior, cholesterol level, and blood pressure. The assessment of eligibility required the collection and analysis of blood, measurement of blood pressure, and an interview to characterize smoking behavior. Nearly 362,000 men were screened to find the 12,866 men enrolled into the trial; including women might have produced valuable information, but at a substantial additional cost.

## Subgroup Analysis

In the context of any clinical study, an *interaction* is a relationship in which the response to treatment is moderated or influenced by some other variable or variables. The variable may be a demographic characteristic (e.g., gender) or some other baseline characteristic or variable (e.g., non-smoker). An interaction effect is said to exist when the treatment effect differs depending on which status of a demographic or baseline variable a person exhibits—such as being a woman or man. A *qualitative interaction* is one in which the direction or sign of the relationship depends on the value assumed by the demographic or baseline variable of interest (e.g., one in which the treatment effect is beneficial for males but is harmful for females). A *quantitative interaction* is one in which the sign or direction of the relationship is the same, but the magnitude of the effect is different. A *subgroup analysis* in this context is any comparison of treatments within a given population, using one or more demographic or baseline characteristics to define subgroups. The characteristics of interest here are those having to do with *biological differences* associated with gender, race, ethnicity, and age (IOM, 1993a).

Most of the researchers who design and analyze clinical trials are skeptical of any observed differences in treatment effects among demographic subgroups unless there is a clear scientific rationale (grounded in biological differences) or until the differential outcome has been replicated in other studies. The underlying assumption is that treatments that work well in one demographic subgroup are likely to work well in another, unless there is a biologically plausible reason for believing otherwise. This argues for the inclusion of women, but not necessarily for the proactive recruitment of sufficient numbers to be able to perform meaningful subgroup analyses. Nevertheless, in the interests of adding to the knowledge of whether there are any unsuspected differences by gender (or other key demographic characteristics), the committee believes that examination of subgroups—where feasible given the number of people enrolled in each subgroup—is to be encouraged.

## Alternatives to Clinical Trials

Strategies other than clinical trials are available to help devise hypotheses about the differential response of men and women to medical interventions. These strategies may be significantly less costly than large-scale clinical trials that include sufficient numbers of men and women to detect gender differences in response. Meta-analysis is one such strategy that is inherently inexpensive and particularly useful for detecting subtle associations between interventions and outcomes and between demographic characteristics and drug effects (IOM, 1993a). Outcomes research, which involves systematic study of the health impact of an intervention, is another such strategy. Pharmacoepidemiologic research is a specific type of outcomes research designed specifically for the study of drug effects in user populations.

Meta-analysis refers to a set of quantitative techniques for combining data from different studies of the same or similar phenomena. From information obtained from each study, a synthesis is made that may produce a much stronger conclusion than any of the studies by themselves can provide. Meta-analysis can be used by clinical investigators to detect significant differences between treatment and control groups where sample sizes in individual studies were too small to allow the detection of statistically significant effects. At the same time, meta-analysis may reveal through averaging that an effect that appeared to be significant in one study is actually less significant. Meta-analysis also allows investigators to detect contradictions or discrepancies among groups of studies. Faced with a collection of studies in a particular area of research, investigators may analyze and compare subgroups of studies with, for example, divergent findings to detect mediating factors of study design, treatment, context, measurement, or analysis that otherwise may not have appeared noteworthy (Pillemer and Light, 1980). The utility of meta-analysis techniques depends on assumptions made about similarities among grouped studies.

The pharmaceutical industry has recently placed renewed emphasis on the use of nonexperimental, observational, epidemiologic techniques—or pharmacoepidemiologic techniques—as alternatives (and sometimes complements) to randomized controlled clinical trials. Postmarketing surveillance is one of several pharmacoepidemiologic techniques employed to study the effects of drugs in uncontrolled, "real life" settings, and in larger numbers of people than can be included in the drug development process. Pharmacoepidemiologic studies avoid some of the important shortcomings of clinical trials, namely the introduction of intervention and observation effects, and the exclusion of effects resulting from the usage of concomitant medications, presence of other illnesses, and lack of patient compliance (Tilson, 1993).

The coincident revolutions in computer technology and health care management have yielded an important new resource for pharmacoepidemiology: large, automated, multipurpose databases of patient information collected by health maintenance organizations. In some cases (e.g., Group Health Cooperative of Puget Sound in Seattle, Washington), these databases contain medical records for as many 300,000 persons in a particular geographic area. Such large databases permit the epidemiologist to collect information on all drug exposures (because the databases include bills or records of disbursement of drugs from pharmacies) and all major medical outcomes (because the databases include bills or statements of diagnoses from clinics), and to take into account major stratifying variables (Tilson, 1993). Where calculated rates of adverse events among users tend to unreliable, largely as a result of underreporting and differential reporting, a structured epidemiologic study can be a powerful tool for quantitatively studying unexpected adverse events.

Although pharmacoepidemiologic studies are generally less costly than clinical trials, these studies can also be complex and expensive, particularly if the risk of an adverse event is small (and the population needed to detect events therefore large); if the event itself is subtle (and monitoring is complex); and if the period of potential risk is long (and the population must be studied for a long time) (Tilson, 1993). However, in cases in which it is impossible or unacceptable to conduct randomized controlled clinical trials (e.g., in persons dying of HIV disease), these studies provide a critical alternative.

Recently, the pharmaceutical industry has experimented with new techniques designed to expedite and enhance the results of drug development.

One of these techniques, which may be useful in detecting differential responses to drugs between men and women (as well as other subgroup differences), is the pharmacokinetic screen. The *pharmacokinetics* of a drug refer to the drug's absorption, distribution, and metabolism in the body, as well as the drug's excretion from the body. A *pharmacokinetic screen* is a technique that can be used during drug development to infer the influence of demographic factors such as age and gender on pharmacokinetics and to suggest the likelihood that a drug-drug or drug-disease interaction will (or will not) occur. The screening process involves the analysis of drug levels in members of specific subgroups at designated points (e.g., before and after dosage) throughout the course of a Phase III trial. Conducting a pharmacokinetic screen during drug development adds little extra cost to the development process, because the necessary data are collected from patients already participating in trials.

## CONCLUSIONS AND RECOMMENDATIONS

In general, the committee's findings are compatible with the NIH mandate for broader inclusion of women and ethnic and racial groups in clinical studies, but with some important caveats, summarized here. The difficult policy issues about including women in clinical studies do not arise when a disease or condition is exclusive to men. Clearly, they do not arise when the study is based on administrative records such as insurance claims, because it is relatively easy to sample patients of both genders. Instead, they attend studies that require large resources to administer and collect new data. For these reasons we focus our concluding remarks on clinical trials of treatment effects for diseases that affect both women and men—namely treatment trials.

The committee finds that the weight of scientific evidence, as well as practical considerations, supports the inclusion of both genders—and indeed all kinds of demographic subgroups—wherever possible. The most compelling scientific reasons for exclusion are found in investigations of diseases, conditions, or risk factors (including behavior) that are highly concentrated in a single gender. Ethical concerns such as an incapacity to give valid informed consent can provide compelling reasons for exclusion irrespective of the presence of scientific reasons, but these are discussed elsewhere in this report.

This is not to say that there are no significant gender-specific diseases or treatment effects, nor do we mean to argue that sufficient attention has been paid to the possibility of gender-specific differences. We support the need to examine these issues systematically where they are based on well-grounded scientific hypotheses, and we support attempts to encourage scientists and clinicians to consider and pursue such gender-related hypotheses. We also acknowledge, however, that most treatments and most diseases do *not* differ significantly in their effect by gender. This observation reinforces rather than reduces the justification for a principle of inclusion: if indeed most treatment effects in the setting of treatment trials do not differ by gender, then it is reasonable for treatment trials to include both genders.

Scientific considerations suggest that the overarching principle should be inclusion. Some would argue that excluding women is justified in a trial where there is no anticipated difference in how women and men respond to a treatment but where the disease is less common among women. These arguments rest on a false assumption that women's presence diminishes homogeneity and thereby lessens the ability to observe the main effect of the treatment (i.e., whether the treatment is effective for any subject). Person-years of follow-up are person-years of follow-up whether they are female or male years, *unless* the researchers have plausible hypotheses about gender differences in response. And if they *do* have convincing hypotheses about qualitative gender-specific differences, then this too argues for including both genders, but in sufficient numbers to test for gender-specific results.

When there are no anticipated treatment effects by gender, however, a policy that requires scientists to include sufficient representation of both genders to permit subgroup analyses would require, at a minimum, that clinical trials significantly increase their size (to detect the main effect in each group) and proportionately increase their expenses. The committee has two concerns in this case, one about the meaning of any information gained by "data dredging," and the other about the appropriateness of spending finite research dollars to satisfy requirements that have little possibility of producing useful information.

The NIH Revitalization Act of 1993 (P.L. 103-43) appears to be based on an intent that is consistent with the principles stated in this chapter, with one important exception. Before excusing a clinical trial from implementing a design with sufficient power to detect subgroup interactions, the act requires investigators to produce "substantial scientific data" of no gender (or race or ethnic) differences. Although the committee agrees with the intent, we believe that this criterion is too extreme given the nature of scientific evidence. Instead, we would suggest a requirement that applicants for funding provide a continuing review of the evidence pertaining to gender-specific effects, along with an assessment of the sample sizes (and costs) that would be necessary to support subgroup analyses.

The committee is concerned that the policy has gone too far by insisting that each and every clinical trial be designed to ensure sufficient numbers of subjects of both genders to permit subgroup analyses. In an era of concern about the nation's resources, and about expenditures on health in particular, we argue that a trial-by-trial application of this requirement is neither good policy nor good science. Clinical trials should include both genders, but requiring scientists to enroll sufficient numbers to ensure the statistical power to detect unsuspected and implausible gender differences would produce little additional information at greatly increased cost. Instead, mechanisms are needed at the national level to ensure that more attention is paid to questions of justice and gender in the setting of research agendas, and at the study level to encourage the appropriate consideration of gender-related effects in clinical studies. The specific actions we suggest to accomplish these goals are discussed in Chapter 8; our general recommendations are as follows:

**The committee recommends that NIH commission a study to identify known gender differences in drug response.**

**The committee recommends that investigators be attentive to factors associated with possible gender differences in drug response and design their studies accordingly. Further, NIH should commission a study that will assist investigators in their effort to detect such differences.**

**The committee recommends that investigators avoid exclusions based on demographic characteristics.**

**The committee recommends that investigators proposing research involving human subjects provide a reasonable review of the evidence and plausibility of gender-specific effects relevant to their research, and that studies be required to be designed with sufficient power to detect subgroup differences only when such a review indicates that such a design is warranted. When there is no information concerning possible gender differences, however, the investigator should, when feasible, include both genders in sufficient number to detect differences.**

Strategies other than clinical trials, (e.g., surveillance techniques) are available to help devise hypotheses about the differential response of men and women to medical interventions. These strategies may be significantly less costly than large-scale clinical trials that include sufficient numbers of men and women to detect gender differences in response.

**The committee recommends that NIH assist investigators in this effort by: (1) identifying, developing, and disseminating alternative methods for detecting or formulating hypotheses about gender differences and (2) providing guidance for the use of these methods by investigators and initial review groups.**

# REFERENCES

Bush, T.L. 1992. Feminine forever revisited: Menopausal hormone therapy in the 1990s. *Journal of Women's Health* 1(1):1-4.

CDPRG (Coronary Drug Project Research Group). 1973. The Coronary Drug Project: Design, Methods and Baseline Results. American Heart Monograph No. 38, New York: American Heart Association.

Everitt, D., and Avorn, J. 1986. Drug prescribing for the elderly. *Archives of Internal Medicine* 1986:146(12):2393-2396.

Finucane, F.F., Madans, J.H., Bush, T.L., Wolf, P.H., and Kleian, J.C. 1993. Decreased risk of stroke among postmenopausal hormone users: Results from a national cohort. *Archives of Internal Medicine* 153:73-79.

GAO (General Accounting Office). 1992. Women's Health: FDA Needs to Ensure More Study of Gender Differences in Prescription Drug Testing. GAO/HRD-93-17. Washington, D.C.: GAO.

Gillette, J.R. 1977. Factors that affect drug concentration in maternal plasma. Pp. 35-77 in Handbook of Teratology, Vol. 3, J.G. Wilson and F.C. Fraser, eds. New York: Plenum.

Horton, J.A., ed. 1992. The Women's Health Data Book. Washington, D.C.: The Jacobs Institute of Women's Health.

Hytten, F.E., and Chamberlain, G. 1980. *Clinical Physiology in Obstetrics*. Oxford, England: Blackwell.

IOM (Institute of Medicine). 1993a. Inclusion of Women in Clinical Trials: Policies for Population Subgroups. Washington, D.C.: National Academy Press.

IOM (Institute of Medicine). 1993b. *Women and Drug Development*. Report of a workshop, Forum on Drug Development. Washington, D.C.: National Academy Press.

Jensvold, M.F., Reed, K., Jarrett, D.B., and Hamilton, J.A. 1992. Menstrual-cycle related depressive symptoms treated with variable antidepressant dosage. *Journal of Women's Health* 1(2):109-115.

Matthews, K.A., Meilahn, E., Kuller, L.H., Kelsey, S.F., Caggiula, A.W., and Wing, R.R. 1989. Menopause and risk factors for coronary heart disease. *New England Journal of Medicine* 321(10):641-646.

Mattison, D. 1986. Physiological variations in pharmacokinetics during pregnancy. Pp. 37-102 in Drug and Chemical Action in Pregnancy, S. Fabro and A.R. Scialli, eds. New York: Marcel Dekker, Inc.

Mattison, D.R. 1990. Transdermal drug absorption during pregnancy. *Clinical Obstetrics and Gynecology* 33:718-727.

Mattison, D.R., and Jelovsek, F.R. 1991. Environmental and occupational exposures. Pp. 91-109 in Reproductive Risks and Prenatal Diagnosis, M.I. Evans, ed. Norwalk, Conn.: Appleton & Lange.

Mattison, D.R., Malek, A., and Cistola, C. 1992. Physiological Adaptations to Pregnancy: Impact on Pharmacokinetics. Pp. 81-96 in Pediatric Pharmacology: Therapeutic Principles in Practice, 2nd ed., J. Aranda and S.J. Yaffe, eds. Philadelphia: W.B. Saunders.

McGrath, E., Keita, G.P., Strickland, B.R., and Russo, N.F. (eds). 1990. Women and Depression: Risk Factors and Treatment Issues, Final Report of the American Psychological Association's National Task Force on Women and Depression. Washington, D.C.: American Psychological Association.

Mosher, W.D. 1990. Contraceptive practice in the United States, 1982-1988. *Family Planning Perspectives* 22:198-205.

Multiple Risk Factor Trial Group. 1977. Statistical design considerations in the NHLI Multiple Risk Factor Intervention Trial (MRFIT). *Journal of Chronic Disease* 30:261-275.

Nabulsi, A.A., Folsom, A.R., White, A., Patsch, W., Heiss, G., Wu, K.K., and Szklo, M. 1993.

Association of hormone-replacement therapy with various cardiovascular risk factors in postmenopausal women. *New England Journal of Medicine* 328(15):1069-1075.

National Center for Health Statistics. 1985. Current Estimates from National Health Interview Survey. Vital and Health Statistics. Atlanta, Ga.: National Center for Health Statistics, Centers for Disease Control, Series 10, No. 160.

National Center for Health Statistics. 1993. Chartbook on Health Data on Older Americans, 1992. Atlanta, Ga.: National Center for Health Statistics, Centers for Disease Control, Series 3, No. 29.

National Medical Expenditure Survey. 1987. Prescribed Medicines: A Summary of Use and Expenditures by Medicare Beneficiary. Dept. H, 45, Research Findings 3.

National Women's Health Resource Center. 1990. Forging a Women's Health Research Agenda. Washington, D.C.: National Women's Health Resource Center.

NIA (National Institute on Aging). 1992. Bound for Good Health: A Collection of Age Pages. Bethesda, Md.: NIA.

NIH (National Institute of Health). 1993. Consensus Development Panel on Triglyceride, High-Density Lipoprotein, and Coronary Heart Disease. Triglyceride, high-density lipoprotein, and coronary heart disease. *Journal of the American Medical Association* 269(4):505-510.

NIH (National Institutes of Health). 1992. Opportunities for Research on Women's Health. Proceedings of a conference in Hunt Valley, Md., Sept. 4-6, 1991. Bethesda, Md.: NIH.

NIH (National Institutes of Health). Advisory Committee on Women's Health Issues. 1988. Women's Health Issues Research Report, FY 1985-1987. Bethesda, Md.

NRC (National Research Council). 1993. Pesticides in the Diets of Infants and Children. Washington, D.C.: National Academy Press.

Olshansky, S.J., Carnes, B.A., and Cassel, C.K. 1993. The aging of the human species. *Scientific American* (April):46-52.

Pelkonen, O. 1980. Biotransformation of xenobiotics by the fetus. *Pharmacology and Therapeutics* 10:26.

Pillemer, D.B., and Light, R.J. 1980. Synthesizing outcomes: How to use research evidence from many studies. *Harvard Education Review* 50:176-195.

Rodin, J., and Ickovics, J.R. 1990. Women's health: Review and research agenda as we approach the 21st century. *American Psychologist* (September):1018-1034.

Silvaggio, T., and Mattison, D.R. 1993. Comparative approach to toxicokinetics, In: Occupational and Environmental Reproductive Hazards: A Guide for Clinicians, M. Paul, ed. Baltimore, Md.: Williams & Wilkins.

Stampfer, M.J., Coditz, G.A., Willett, W.C., Manson, J.E., Rosner, B., Spaizer, F.E., and Hennekens, C.H. 1991. Postmenopausal estrogen therapy and cardiovascular disease: Ten year follow-up from the nurse's health study. *New England Journal of Medicine* 325(11):756-762.

Tanner, L.A., Baum, C., Prela, C.-M., and Kennedy, D.L. 1989. Spontaneous adverse reporting in the elderly for 1985. *Journal of Geriatric Drug Therapy* 3(3):31-54.

Teichmann, A.T. 1990. Influence of oral contraceptives on drug therapy. *American Journal of Obstetrics and Gynecology* 163:2208-2213.

Tilson, H. 1993. Observational studies making an overdue and much needed comeback: Alternatives and complements to randomization. In: Clinical Trials and Statistics: Proceedings of a Symposium. Washington, D.C.: National Academy Press.

U.S. Bureau of the Census. 1992. Statistical Abstract of the United States: 1992 (112th ed.). Washington, D.C.

Weatherall, D.J., et al., eds. 1988. Oxford Textbook of Medicine, Volume 2. New York: Oxford University Press.

Yonkers, K.A., Kando, J.C., Cole, J.O., and Blumenthal, S. 1992. Gender differences in pharmacokinetics and pharmacodynamics of psychotropic medication. *American Journal of Psychiatry* 149(5):587-595.

# 5

# Social and Ethical Considerations

The process of clinical research takes place in a social, ethical, and legal context that shapes and constrains the pursuit of science. The governments, foundations, and corporations that provide financial support for scientific research also provide ethical guidelines for its conduct. Negotiation and maintenance of boundaries between scientific and nonscientific spheres is constant and often problematic. It is not clear, however, that the goals of each sphere are necessarily incompatible; good science and good public policy can be pursued in tandem, although not without some effort. NIH's legislative mandate to ensure greater gender equity in clinical studies can be viewed as an explicit attempt to create a balance between the goals of science and those of public policy.

This chapter examines the ways in which the social and ethical constraints affecting the way science operates present challenges to the achievement of equity in clinical studies. The "legal" world—as it is more narrowly construed to mean federal policies and liability issues—will be discussed in the following chapter.

The social context may explain the differential treatment of men and women as scientific research participants, which raises the question of whether science is truly "value neutral" with respect to gender. Similarly, in a society composed of different races, ethnicities, and economic backgrounds, unconscious biases may render those of lesser power and status "invisible" to those of greater power and status. This invisibility can affect the conduct of scientific research in important ways, such as a lack of investigation into diseases that are pervasive among certain racial and ethnic groups, or a tendency to focus on the reproductive capability of women while ignoring that of men. Finally, these influences have significant practical implications for the design of research studies, for recruitment and retention strategies in diverse populations, and for logistical and cost issues. There is a particular concern for the potential exploitation of disadvantaged individuals and communities who are ascribed lower status and power in our society; the principal protection against this possibility is the informed consent process.

## SCIENCE AND OBJECTIVITY

As in all scientific endeavors, clinical studies seek to achieve results that are unbiased by the preconceptions or preferences of investigators, staff, or study participants. This does not mean that the conduct of science is necessarily objective. Many of the principles and methods of the conduct of science can be viewed as precautions to protect the objectivity of the results from a process that is inherently subjective (NAS, 1989). This issue is at the core of many debates about the underlying biases within scientific processes.

Does science reflect the society and culture in which it evolves? For example, is it permeated by the biases related to gender, race, or ethnicity that operate in the broader culture? For some the answer would be no, that science produces a higher, universal "truth" that will always be triumphant (Nagel, 1961; Popper, 1981). These commentators rely on a rational model of the scientific process in which deductive reasoning and observational refutation provide the basis for "objective" results (Popper, 1981).

By contrast, other scholars have argued that science does reflect the culture in which it evolves, including its biases. In the literature on the sociology of knowledge and the history and philosophy of science, for example, Mannheim (1936) and Kuhn (1970) posit that we can only relate to any experience on the basis of our social and historical understanding. In other words, some subjectivity is unavoidable:

> Observation and experience can and must drastically restrict the range of admissible belief, else there would be no science . . . but an apparently arbitrary element, compounded of personal and historical accident, is always a formative ingredient of the beliefs espoused by a given scientific community at a given time [Kuhn, 1970].

Kuhn (1970) maintains that "normal science" tends to present a conservative, status quo approach toward knowledge, not because scientists are entrenched in powerful social positions, but because "fundamental novelties . . . are necessarily subversive of its basic commitments." He sees dramatic revolutions in scientific thinking as the result of a profound shift in the basic assumptions and body of knowledge considered applicable to specific scientific problems, labeling this process a "paradigm shift." So, for example, the works of Einstein and Copernicus were revolutionary precisely because they forced such paradigm shifts: scientists had to discard the basic assumptions that formed the foundation of their work, substituting new ideas and examining new evidence.

Similarly, Mannheim (1936) argues that individual "thinkers" operate in an inherited context, seeking to elaborate on that context or to substitute other contexts that deal more adequately with new challenges. Scientific observation is not an isolated act but one that is "colored by values and collective-unconscious, volitional impulses" that permeate not only science but politics, justice, religion, journalism, division of labor, and language.

This perspective on science has led some observers to argue that scientific knowledge is fundamentally biased by context and social values. That this view currently represents a consensus is suggested by the conclusions of the National Academy of Sciences Committee on the Conduct of Science (NAS, 1989):

> Scientific knowledge emerges from a process that is intensely human, a process marked by its full share of human virtues and limitations. . . . Many people think of scientific research as a routine, cut-and-dried process. They associate the nature of scientific knowledge with the process of deriving it and conclude that research is as objective and unambiguous as scientific results. The reality is much different. Researchers continually have to make difficult decisions about how to do their work and how to present their work to others. Scientists have a large body of knowledge that they can use in making these decisions. Yet, much of this knowledge is not the product of scientific investigation, but instead involves value-laden judgment, personal desires, and even a researcher's personality and style.

These debates about the observational biases, processes, and the conservatism of science are basic to many of the legal and ethical issues regarding inclusion of women in clinical studies. We turn next to these more specific applications.

## QUESTIONS OF GENDER

Bem (1993), writing on the issues of male bias and male norms in scientific and political discourse, offers a useful analogy to explain the power and pervasiveness of biases. The basic, hidden assumptions involving gender—so basic as to be transparent—are "lenses" through which people perceive, conceive, and discuss social and scientific reality. It is important to look *at* these lenses in order to understand their consequences, instead of looking *through* them. Two types of gender-based assumptions—or lenses— seem particularly relevant to this report:

1. *Male bias* refers to the "observer bias" present in scientific inquiry when scientist-observers adopt male perspectives.

2. *Male norm* refers to the tendency to perceive men's identity and experience as the characterization or standard of what it is to be a person and to portray female differences, where they occur, as "deviant."

These lenses can operate independently or simultaneously and can affect observations regardless of the gender of the scientist-observer (women scientists can adopt the cultural values of male biases).

## Male Bias

The observer effect is a well-studied and accepted phenomenon in the social sciences, but it is more invisible in the biological and clinical sciences, which are viewed as value-neutral. In all scientific fields, however, the theories proposed, questions posed, and data collected are subject to this observer effect. As male bias affects interpretation of information about females, so too do other biases affect the interpretation of information about other less powerful groups, including racial and ethnic groups, the poor, the elderly, and homosexuals.

As an historical example of male bias, Bem (1993) cites the nineteenth century scientific theories that were used to justify the lack of education for women. Arguing from the physical law of conservation of energy, Edward Clarke reasoned that the reproductive capacity of women, especially women during menstruation, would be irreparably harmed by education because thinking would detract from the energy needed by the uterus. As evidence of this harm, Clarke pointed out that educated women had a lower birth rate. While these arguments can be dismissed on the basis of faulty logic and false premises, they illustrate a bias toward finding evidence that women are inferior or legitimately kept from some activities. Bleier (1988) offers a more modern example in the field of neuroscience: major scientific journals tend to publish research supporting the prevailing wisdom that there are biological differences in the brains of males and females and to find flaws in research that contradicts this widely held view.

Altekruse and McDermott (1988) provide examples of similar biases in clinical research, arguing that scientific inquiry—were it to fully recognize the differences between men's and women's social roles (and perhaps in their biology)—would differ in several critical areas. For example, the fields of sports medicine, psychiatry, and occupational medicine would focus on different issues if women's recreational and nonrecreational activities and stresses dominated. Indeed, the specialties themselves might have developed differently, focusing on leisure activities instead of "sports," or on the hazards of domestic activities instead of those of the workplace.

These and other critics suggest that mere recognition of potential gender-related differences by male scientists is not enough: what is needed are *female* scientists and physicians, because females in these positions are likely to choose different problems and frame clinical problems differently (Healy, 1991). For example, one study on human immunodeficiency virus (HIV) showed that there are more female participants when the principal investigator or study director is female (Cotton et al., 1993). According to this view, the low number of women scientists, particularly at the upper levels of the research hierarchy, is directly related to the level of women's participation in clinical studies and the amount of attention devoted to women's health concerns. Recent analyses of women's advancement in medical and scientific careers (e.g., by the NIH Office of Research on Women's Health) are also evaluating institutional barriers to women's attainment of coveted positions in these fields.

Arguing from a broader perspective, Belenky et al. (1986) suggest that women's ways of knowing differ importantly from men's. Their interviews suggest that women are more likely than men to use interactive modes to collect information and to trust subjective responses. Applying this line of argument to clinical studies and practice, suppose that obstetrical and gynecological needs were handled by female instead of male practitioners (as had been common in the United States until the eighteenth century). The roles of these physicians and their language might have developed very differently, perhaps concentrating more on trusting the birthing mother's actions and "interacting" with the natural processes under distress, rather than "controlling" the birthing process and "fixing" problems with invasive procedures (Bogdan, 1990).

A final example of male bias in the collection of information is the strong tendency to believe "hard" data that are "objective," even when these data have little clinical relevancy. Stephen Jay Gould (1981) illustrates the consequences of this illusion of objectivity through numbers with a complex story of political and social discrimination against classes of people proven by "science" to be "inferior":

> This . . . is the story of numbers once regarded as surpassing all others in importance—the data of craniometry or the measurement of the skull and its contents. The leaders of craniometry . . . regarded themselves as servants of their numbers, apostles of objectivity. And [their results] confirmed all the common prejudices of comfortable white males—that blacks, women and poor people occupy their subordinate roles by the harsh dictates of nature.

## Male Norm

Male norm refers to the tendency to conceive of men gender neutrally, as persons, rather than to conceive of men in terms of their sex. Thus, men's identity and experience becomes the characterization or standard of what it is to be a human being (DeBruin, 1994). An example is the argument that men make more appropriate research subjects for drug studies because, for example, women have menstrual cycles that produce deviations from the "normal" pattern of drug disposition observable in males. Basic biologic differences between the sexes are valid and relevant for some scientific research, but when male-only studies are regarded as the scientific "ideal" for conducting research (e.g., to ensure homogeneity across the groups being compared), the male physiology becomes the implicit "normal" standard for judging etiology, pathology, and response to intervention. By contrast, female physiology needs to be examined only to the supposed extent that it deviates from the male norm. This can promote the misuse of scientific rationales to justify protectionism and current practices, but it can also compromise subsequent clinical practice by leaving clinicians and patients uncertain about the applicability of research findings to women.

The male norm may play a role in the design of clinical studies that include only men, but that are focused on a disease or condition that affects both genders. These single-gender studies are designed for a number of practical reasons, such as the convenience and availability of a single-gender population for study (e.g., prisons, VA hospitals), or because of an interest in a particular manifestation that occurs more frequently in males (e.g., midlife cardiovascular events). Nevertheless, all-male studies have also occurred when no particular practical or scientific justification is put forward for excluding women, either because the investigators have a conscious preference for studying men or, more likely, because they have been blinded to the need to include women by the male norm gender lens.

Regardless of their motivations, a primary concern raised about male-only clinical studies relates to their external validity and the generalizability of their results to women, who will likely be diagnosed and treated based on the findings of such research. As a case in point, three out of four randomized clinical trials on cholesterol-lowering drugs were conducted using only middle-age men (Muldoon et al., 1990), yet half of the prescriptions for these drugs were written for women over 60 years of age (Wysowski et al., 1990).

Uncertainty of treatment can also lead to wide variation in treatment patterns (Wennberg, 1991). As a result of greater ambiguity in applying the treatment to women, some clinicians may adopt a conservative approach (withholding treatment for women until further evidence is collected), while others may apply a liberal approach (assuming that the study findings can be generalized to all patients). These arguments have even greater cogency when considering children and pregnant women. Ironically, if researchers deliberately avoid these groups because of concerns about harm, they may be placing them at greater risk by withholding a potentially useful treatment.

This tendency to view men's identity and experience as universal—to subscribe to "false universalism," as defined by philosopher Debra DeBruin—may operate in a subconscious fashion. The subtlety and lens-like transparency of false universalism makes it difficult to attribute malice or deliberate intent, but it nevertheless may result in making women "invisible" in a general sense and "deviant" with regard to clinical studies.

## QUESTIONS OF RACE AND ETHNICITY

### The Diversity of Women

Gender is not the only significant difference to which science may be insensitive. There are other important differences among groups that can have a significant impact on health and illness, and have historically received scant or inadequate attention by clinical researchers. A growing body of evidence (*Journal of the American Medical Association* Special Issue on Hispanic Health, 1991; Amaro, 1993; *Annals of Epidemiology* Special Issue on African American Health, 1993; Amaro and Vega, in press), including substantial contributions from scholars of color some of whose work is cited here, indicates that variables such as race, ethnicity, rural and urban background, socioeconomic status, and sexual orientation should be examined in clinical studies.

Recent federal legislation on the inclusion of women and racial and ethnic groups in clinical research has major implications for the investigation of race and ethnicity as explanatory variables in clinical studies. One provision of the recently enacted NIH Revitalization Act requires that clinical research be designed and carried out in a manner that provides valid analyses of whether the variables under study affect women or members of racial and ethnic groups differently than other participants. In order to comply with the intent of the legislation, researchers will have to develop effective outreach, recruitment, and retention strategies and to employ scientific methods that are appropriate and valid for ethnically diverse populations.

This promises to contribute to scientific knowledge on the impact of gender, race, and ethnicity on disease and treatment. It also presents researchers with complex conceptual and methodological challenges, requiring them to clearly define and operationalize race and ethnicity and to show specifically how these variables relate to the research questions under study. In addition, the scientific community must adapt current methods and develop new, more appropriate methods for specific racial and ethnic groups. As a result, methodology becomes a critical factor in determining the risk-benefit ratio for participation and assessing the ethics of conducting such research. To aid researchers in this complex task of inclusion, it may be advisable to draw on the expertise of those researchers who routinely examine the impact of gender, race and ethnicity in their respective fields of research (e.g., social anthropologists, sociologists, social epidemiologists, psychologists, etc.) in order to avail themselves of the most accurate and current conceptualizations and measurements of these variables relevant to their own investigations. The complexity of proper conceptualization and measurement of such variables is treated in the section which follows.

The inclusion of women from diverse racial and ethnic groups therefore confronts each researcher with a set of complex issues that must be addressed and used to inform the research design and approach, including:

- the constructions of race and ethnicity in each research study;
- the specific context and meaning of research within participants' racial and ethnic communities.

Related issues relevant to the recruitment, retention, and the protection of research participants through the informed consent process will be treated in the following section.

## Constructions of Race and Ethnicity

### Biology or Sociology?

Health research, including clinical research, has given little systematic consideration to race and almost none to ethnicity. Even when race is included as a variable under study, investigators generally fail to establish whether race is considered to have a biological or a sociological connection (Gamble and Blustein, 1994; Williams, in press).

Biological constructions of race highlight the impact of genetic characteristics or genotypic differences along racial lines. The genetic model of racial differences has been based on the following assumptions: "(1) race is a valid biological category; (2) the genes which determine race are linked to those that determine health; and (3) the health of a population is largely determined by the biological constitution of the population" (Krieger and Bassett, 1986). This concept of race has been criticized by those who believe that "race is a societally constructed taxonomy that reflects the intersection of biological, cultural, socioeconomic, political, and legal factors, as well as racism" (Williams et al., 1993).

The ways in which race is defined are highly variable and reflect strong sociological influences (Williams et al., 1993; Gamble and Blustein, 1994; Williams, in press). While genetic and biological factors may contribute to racial differences in health and response to certain treatments, these differences may also reflect "habitual behaviors of a social group in response to the constraints of its environment" (Williams et al., 1993). When researchers do not give sufficient attention to understanding when and how biological differences between races are the consequences of differential living conditions, they may draw erroneous conclusions about the role of biology in racial differences (Williams, 1993).

This conceptual confusion has led to varying definitions of race across disciplines and to inconsistencies in the ways national health data systems and health research have defined race and ethnicity (Yu and Liu, 1992; Amaro, 1993; Williams, 1993, in press; Gamble and Blustein, 1994). The most common ways of assessing race have been self-identification and interviewer or provider assessment. The latter relies primarily on skin color, a phenotypic attribute that does not always correspond well to genotypic differences or to self-identification (Gamble and Blustein, 1994; Williams, 1993, in press). Methods of classification have also changed over time and across geographic locations, reflecting arbitrary and inconsistent definitions of race (Hahn, 1992; Gamble and Blustein, 1994; Williams, 1993, in press).

This lack of attention to the conceptualization of race and its assessment leads to inappropriate conclusions in health research. After a thorough review of the use of race in the health services research literature from 1966 to 1990, Williams (1993) concluded that "using race only as an afterthought and/or in a mechanical and a theoretical manner does not shed any light on the ways in which racial differences are built into the institutions of society, and serves only to perpetuate the distortion of social reality." Thus, clinical researchers must pay careful attention to the conceptualization and measurement of race and must provide an explicit rationale for the omission or inclusion of analyses to investigate racial and ethnic differences.

## Faulty Constructions of Ethnicity

The study of ethnic group and subgroup differences in clinical research is embryonic. Researchers rarely consider differences within ethnic subgroups, often inappropriately grouping individuals from different ethnic backgrounds (Amaro, 1993; Lex and Norris, 1994; Yu, 1994; Zambrana, 1994; Williams, 1993, in press). National health data also combines information for Hispanics, Asians and Pacific Islanders, and American Indians and Alaskan Natives, ignoring the vast differences between their subgroups (Yu and Liu, 1992; Amaro, 1993; Williams, 1993, in press; Yu, 1994).

As with race, definitional issues arise in the measurement of ethnicity.

Yu (1994) highlights the complexity of this task with the following questions:

> What should one use as the criteria for defining whether someone is an Asian/Pacific Islander or a member of subgroups of its populations, such as Chinese, Japanese, Filipinos, Hawaiians, Samoans, Guamanians or others? Should the definition be based on ancestry? Self definition of ethnicity? Or interviewer observation of "race," as has occurred in several government surveys prior to 1976?

Despite the conceptual and measurement issues, most scientists who have written on this topic believe that the relationships between race, ethnicity, and health should be investigated. And just as researchers should articulate how race and ethnicity relate to the questions under study, they must also consider how differences in results by race or ethnicity could be explained— not only by biological factors but also by socioeconomic status and other social status characteristics, such as being the direct target of racism (Williams, 1993, in press; Gamble and Blustein, 1994).

Subgroup information must also be disaggregated, however, because there are substantial differences in socioeconomic status, access and utilization of health services, migration, and political history within each racial and ethnic group (Yu and Liu, 1992; Amaro, 1993; Williams, in press; Lex and Norris, 1994; Zambrana, 1994; Gamble and Blustein, 1994).

## One Model of Health Does Not Fit All Groups

Historically, the absence of comprehensive epidemiologic information on the health problems of Asians and Pacific Islanders, American Indians and Alaskan Natives, and Hispanics resulted in placing all these groups into a larger social category of "minorities" (Amaro and Vega, in press). Presumably, to the extent that these groups were exposed to the underclass social conditions faced by African Americans, generalizations derived from that group could be extended to cover other groups as well. Instead, the few dedicated studies of other racial and ethnic groups have demonstrated important differences in mortality and morbidity across and within groups. Consequently, clinical investigators should not employ gross conceptualizations or assessment categories of race and ethnicity based on a "minority" model of health. Categorizations of study samples as "white and nonwhite" or "white and minorities" are scientifically unacceptable. Generalizations from research should be limited to the racial and ethnic groups represented in the study sample, and conclusions regarding racial or ethnic differences (or the lack of such differences) should be limited to groups examined through detailed analyses of differences in each study.

## Context and Meaning of Research in Different Communities

The meaning of participation in clinical research studies for different racial and ethnic groups, including women, has important ethical implications that also affect the scientific validity and merit of the research. For all the major "minority" groups in the United States, participation in research cannot be separated from experiences with a health care system that, according to a former secretary of Health and Human Services, has clearly demonstrated undeniable evidence of discrimination and racism (Sullivan, 1991). Distinctions between health research and health services, which are clearly demarcated for health professionals, are not necessarily clear to the general population. In addition, the history of unethical research that has directly or indirectly led to exploitation, deception, disease, and at times death among diverse ethnic populations adds to the distrust of research in these communities (Brandt, 1985; Jones, 1993; Gamble and Blustein, 1994; Lex and Norris, 1994; Yu, 1994). This history of abuse requires that extraordinary measures be taken to guarantee the ethical treatment of participants from diverse racial and ethnic groups in clinical research (see below).

Each racial and ethnic community has a distinctly different history with regard to research (Gamble and Blustein, 1994; Lex and Norris, 1994; Yu, 1994). Clinical researchers must be familiar with the experience of unethical research in each of these groups in order to ascertain the best methods of addressing distrust and fear and for ensuring appropriate conditions for participation. Among American Indian and Alaskan native peoples, for example, a longstanding history of distrust of government personnel and policies is rooted in an even longer history of disease, coercion, broken contracts, and denial of basic rights (Lex and Norris, 1994). In an effort to protect native peoples from potential abuse, the Indian Health Service has developed detailed guidelines to obtain informed consent for certain invasive procedures, especially those pertinent to reproduction (Lex and Norris, 1994).

The infamous case of the Tuskegee syphilis study conducted by the U.S. Public Health Service, in which 400 poor African American sharecroppers from Macon County, Alabama, infected with syphilis, were denied treatment when treatment options became available, has come to be symbolic of the racism within U.S. medicine and research in particular (Brandt, 1985; Jones, 1993; Gamble and Blustein, 1994). Accounts of unethical and cruel treatment of African Americans as research subjects continues to instill distrust of the medical profession and to affect participation in research and health promotion and intervention efforts (Gamble and Blustein, 1994).

Among Hispanics, women have often been the target of the most blatant unethical research and medical practices. In the early 1960s, poor women in Puerto Rico served as some of the first subjects of experiments with birth control pills, in part because of a lack of legal protection regarding drug testing (Yu, 1994). A study conducted in 1969 in Austin, Texas, told poor Mexican American women that they had been provided with contraceptives, when in fact many of the subjects received placebos; those who became pregnant and requested abortions were denied such services (Adams and Cown, 1972). Such research practices are indicative of a broader climate of unethical medical practices and violations of the reproductive rights of poor women and women from diverse racial and ethnic groups (Rodriguez-Trias, 1976; Gamble and Blustein, 1994). For example, public health fertility control campaigns targeted to increase the use of sterilization among women in Puerto Rico have resulted in inappropriate and uninformed use of this procedure (Presser, 1965; Scrimshaw and Pasquariella, 1970; Vasquez-Calzada, 1973; Rodriguez-Trias, 1976; Schensul et al., 1982).

The legacy of mistrust toward research among Asian and Pacific Islander populations is just as profound but distinctly different from that of the groups discussed above. The history of unethical research with this population includes U.S.-funded research conducted in the countries of origin, as well as the overall oppressive political conditions to which some Asian and Pacific Islander populations have been subjected. An example provided by Yu (1994) is the involuntary radiation exposure of the inhabitants of the Pacific atoll of Eniwetok (now part of the Marshall Islands) as a result of U.S. nuclear testing. These experiences have contributed to distrust of researchers and other individuals perceived, accurately or not, to be "government" representatives.

## RECRUITMENT AND RETENTION ISSUES

### Feasibility, Logistics, and Cost

Under some circumstances, investigators who wish to recruit and retain women in their studies may encounter problems related to feasibility, logistics, and cost. The NIH Revitalization Act specifically discounts the issue of cost in its requirements for investigators to increase the representation of these groups in their studies, yet investigators will need practical guidance in order to comply with the mandate. Some of these problems may apply to women in general; others are relevant primarily to poor women or to women in racial or ethnic groups. Taken together, however, these practical issues may limit the extent to which equity in research can be achieved, and they may prompt investigators to request exemptions from requirements for inclusiveness.

The feasibility of recruiting and retaining participants for clinical studies depends on the number of women in the reference population and their characteristics in relation to the study. If eligible women are rare relative to men, or if eligible women in an ethnic, socioeconomic, or age group of interest are relatively rare in comparison with affluent young white women, a greater effort will be needed to identify and attract them.

The feasibility of studying women is also affected by social conditions that may limit the personal autonomy of women. For example, women may have less flexibility than men regarding lifestyle or keeping appointments during work hours. Personal safety may also be a greater concern with respect to evening appointments, which would require provision of transportation, security guards, and the like. Arranging child care during clinic appointments may be more of a problem when studying women than when dealing with men.

For situations in which menstrual cycle variation or other reproductive variables are related to the issues under study, the feasibility of the study will depend on the ability to schedule or plan around this variability. This may increase recruitment costs (to find enough women with the right reproductive or hormonal status) or increase sample sizes (to balance reproductive or hormonal status within the study population). The most extreme version of this problem arises when all women in their reproductive years are considered to be inappropriate study participants because of potential harm to future offspring (see Chapter 7). If gender is thought to be a modifier of the effects or pathways under study, leading to an interest in studying men and women or subgroups of men and women separately, then an inclusive study will have a larger sample size (i.e., enough in each subgroup) than a study in which one or more subgroup is excluded to achieve homogeneity.

## Outreach and Access

The factors that motivate women to participate in clinical studies—particularly women from diverse racial and ethnic groups, and the elderly and the poor—may be different from those that apply to men. Similarly, the channels of influence whereby women are persuaded to enter and remain in clinical studies may also be culture- or gender-specific. Achieving the goal of a diverse study population may require investigators to develop and implement gender-specific recruitment programs. This could require special or different staffing (e.g., elderly women may be the best people to recruit elderly women into studies) and costly duplication of certain aspects of recruitment for each special population.

## Community Attitudes Towards Research

Decisions regarding appropriateness of individual participation in clinical studies can be influenced by a communal perception of risk and benefit, leading to an overlay of motivation or resistance based on group or community membership. For example, peer pressure or solidarity within a group may enhance an individual's desire to participate in a project that would benefit the group, or to refrain from participating even though personally willing to participate. An example of community attitudes favoring participation of women in a study might be a grassroots movement in favor of participation in a study of breast cancer, a high-profile condition affecting a high proportion of women. An example of attitudes fostering resistance might be fears of African American women about participating in research based on stories of covert sterilizations in the past or the exploitation of African American men in the Tuskegee study.

### Appropriateness of Participation

Any discussion of the participation of women in clinical studies assumes that this is a good thing—that is, that participation in research is beneficial, to society if not to the individual, and that it is appropriate for researchers to solicit participation from individuals in the population at large. The informed consent process (see below) is intended to allow anyone who so wishes to decline or drop out of participation, but there may be some situations in which it is inappropriate, in principle, to request their participation.

For example, is there a threshold standard of living that should be met before it is ethical to solicit a woman's participation in a research study? Does the answer to this question differ according to the level of direct benefit the individual could derive from study participation? That is, is it appropriate to solicit the participation of economically disadvantaged or socially marginal individuals when the study provides a treatment that would otherwise be unavailable to them? This would mean either that there is no placebo condition or that even the placebo condition is an improvement over the care she would otherwise receive. Conversely, is it inappropriate to recruit poor, inner-city women into a study that will benefit society but that will cost them money and time, possibly jeopardize their work performance, and not offer a reasonable assurance of health benefit? Is the obligation to serve society through participation in studies one that accrues only to those for whom society is meeting the minimum need for food, clothing, and shelter? By this reasoning, is research participation one way that persons who owe a debt to society can pay this debt? The committee raises these questions in order to highlight the potential difference between participant and investigator perceptions of justice in clinical studies.

## PROTECTION OF RESEARCH PARTICIPANTS

### Potential for Exploitation

The history of unethical research and broken social contracts with racial and ethnic groups in the United States provides the context for understanding the importance of ensuring ethical practices in clinical research with women in these groups. Because of the lower status ascribed to ethnic populations, especially women in these groups, they are especially at risk for abusive and exploitative research practices. Clinical research with these populations must clearly articulate safeguards for the ethical treatment of participants.

There has always been a tension between, on the one hand, the investigator's need to recruit and retain study participants and, on the other hand, the study participants' right to uncoerced involvement in and free withdrawal from a study at any time. The issue of diversity may further strain the already delicate balance between these two ends: in light of the NIH mandate, the investigator now stands to gain or lose directly in accordance with his or her success in recruiting a diverse study sample. The gain, if in compliance, may be a higher priority for funding or the ability to receive continuation funds. The penalty for noncompliance may be losing research funds. It will be the investigator's and the IRB's responsibility to see that the needs and rights of the participants are balanced against the desirability of including them in the study. One of the most important safeguards for protection of human subjects is informed consent.

### Informed Consent Process

Central to the informed consent process are the requirements that a competent person be given the information necessary for a full understanding of the risks and benefits involved in participating in a research study, and that no coercion or manipulation is used to obtain the potential participant's permission. The informed consent process may become more complex in light of the issues discussed in the preceding sections, such as community attitudes toward research and the legacy of historical exploitation. Monetary compensation for participation in clinical research might be considered an undue influence in any potential subject population; the poorer the population, the more likely it is that such compensation might render poor women vulnerable to disproportionate experimentation (Yu, 1994). Similarly, the real or perceived increased access to health services provided by participation in clinical research may offer relatively more incentive for poor women to participate in experimental treatments than would be the case for other groups.

Although access to participation is desirable, therefore, it is also important to ensure that all potential participants understand the risks and limitations of participating in clinical research. This of course is a concern with
all human subjects; the process of informed consent was developed precisely to ensure that participants receive and understand such information.
In some of the populations of concern here, however, the process of informed consent is more complex than in other groups.

Insofar as the ability to comprehend complicated information depends
on literacy, education, and proficiency in English, for example, it is questionable whether current methods for obtaining informed consent are adequate for many participants from racial and ethnic groups, especially the
poor and recent immigrants (Hurh and Kim, 1982). Valid consent also depends on the investigator's willingness, efforts, and commitment to convey
information in language the participant can understand. Current guidelines
for informed consent are not uniform from institution to institution; some
do not require that written informed consent forms be provided in the participant's
native or dominant language. The more usual practice is to supply a literal
verbal translation of the form or a translation of its major points, by a
translator who may or may not be a member of the research team. This type
of translation can introduce bias and inconsistency into the informed consent process.

Another problem of informed consent that affects immigrant populations and those who have lived under oppressive political regimes is the
lack of understanding of basic human rights as defined in this country (Yu,
1994). Those who have lived in societies where torture and government
coercion are common may fear retaliation for participating or not participating. In addition, social status may unknowingly exert undue influence on an
individual's decision to take part in a clinical study. Yu (1994) reports that
some Asian and Pacific Islander populations are influenced to sign consent
forms because the person who asked for their participation is considered
credible and not because they understand the risks involved.

## CONCLUSIONS AND RECOMMENDATIONS

Within the scientific community, there is no consensus concerning whether
scientific objectivity can be achieved. Some scientists believe that the research process cannot easily be disentangled from the social world within
which it is conducted. Societies stratified by gender, race, ethnicity, and
socioeconomic status provide different "lenses" through which to see and
understand social and scientific reality. These unconscious biases may permeate the entire scientific research process, influencing the research topics
selected, the definition and operationalization of concepts examined, the
study design, the method of data collection employed, and the research

participants chosen for inclusion. Furthermore, such unconscious assumptions contribute to the view that men's physical makeup and experiences are the standard by which to measure and compare women's; to the extent that women's experiences differ from the established male norm, they may be categorized as deviant. These biases impede the progress of the scientific enterprise and produce findings that are not valid for large segments of the population.

**The committee recommends that NIH and IRBs engage in educational efforts that will ensure that investigators are aware of such gender biases and that studies are equitably conceived and designed with respect to gender.**

One way to reduce the influence of such gender biases may be to have a greater number of women scientists active in the research enterprise, through, for example, identification and removal of any institutional barriers to their increased participation. The perspectives they bring to bear may differ markedly from those of their male colleagues, thus aiding in the dissolution of unwarranted and inaccurate assumptions about women in the research enterprise.

**The committee recommends that NIH continue its efforts to encourage women of all racial and ethnic groups to become scientific researchers and to assume positions of authority within the scientific hierarchy.**

Variables such as race, ethnicity, and socioeconomic status can affect health outcomes. The lack of attention to or inadequate conceptualization and measurement of these variables in clinical studies has resulted in findings that are inapplicable to particular racial, ethnic, and socioeconomic groups. For example, in order to accurately determine the effects of race on health and treatment outcomes, it is important to clearly distinguish the biological and sociological components of race. Standard methods of data collection may be inappropriate to certain cultural groups and may need to be modified to ensure that the information obtained is valid and for the risk-benefit ratio to be acceptable. Thus, studies must be planned, designed, and executed to produce valid and generalizable results to the populations under investigation. Investigators and IRBs should utilize the expertise of scholars with experience in studying these populations to avoid the weaknesses evidenced in earlier research.

The history of government-sponsored health research and health care efforts in racial, ethnic, and socioeconomic subgroups has not been unblemished—past unethical treatment has led individuals from these groups to be wary of participation in current studies. Because of the requirements of the NIH Revitalization Act of 1993, researchers now stand to gain or lose support in accordance with their success in recruiting and retaining participants from these same groups, the federal mandate has the potential effect of exacerbating past problems of exploitation. Knowledge of the history of health research in relevant racial or ethnic groups and an awareness of the cultural and political frames of reference employed by the members of these groups will enable researchers to avoid perpetuating the problems.

Informed consent is the primary mechanism for protecting subjects from unethical treatment. NIH, IRBs, and investigators must work together to tailor the consent process so that it will be effective for every group that participates in clinical studies. This entails, for example, both understanding and avoiding what might constitute excessive inducement (monetary or otherwise) for members of a group. If the benefits of research are to accrue to all groups equally, then proper study design and fully informed consent are critical elements to the achievement of that end.

**The committee recommends that NIH commission a study of attitudinal and institutional barriers to participation in research among women, racial and ethnic groups, and the poor.**

**The committee recommends that NIH train IRGs and TEGs and investigators in recruitment and retention issues; part of this training should emphasize methodological and ethical issues in conducting research with women of diverse racial and ethnic groups and poor women.**

**The committee recommends that investigators tailor study designs and recruitment and retention efforts to the specific populations to be included in the study. Investigators must consider the relevance of race, ethnicity, socioeconomic status, and other subgroup variables to their study and develop appropriate definitions, methods, and measurements, to ensure the validity of their research efforts among these groups.**

**The committee recommends that in designing recruitment and consent procedures, investigators be cognizant of concerns and needs of communities that have a history of exploitation or abuse in previous clinical studies. Investigators also must ensure that such information be presented and carefully explained, orally and/or in writing, in the potential participant's preferred language.**

# REFERENCES

Adams and Cown. 1972. The human guinea pig: How we test new drugs, *World* (5 December):21.

Altekruse, J.M., and McDermott, S.W. 1988. Contemporary concerns of women in medicine. Pp. 65-88 in Feminism Within the Science and Health Care Professions: Overcoming Resistance, S.V. Rosser, ed. New York: Pergamon.

Amaro, H. 1993. Women don't get AIDS. They just die from it. Presented at the American Psychological Association Annual Meeting, August 20-24, Toronto, Canada.

Amaro, H., and Vega, W. In press. Health status of Latino population. *Annual Review of Public Health.*

*Annals of Epidemiology.* 1993. Special Issue on African American Health. 3(2).

Belenky, M.F., Clinchy, B.M., Goldberger, N.R., and Tarule, J.M. 1986. *Women's Ways of Knowing: The Development of Self, Voice, and Mind.* New York: Basic Books.

Bem, S.L. 1993. *The Lenses of Gender: Transforming the Debate on Sexual Inequality.* New Haven: Yale University Press.

Bleier, R. 1988. Science and the construction of meaning in the neurosciences. Pp. 91-104 in Feminism Within the Science & Health Care Professions: Overcoming Resistance, S.V. Rosser, ed. New York: Pergamon.

Bogdan, J.C. 1990. Childbirth in America: 1650 to 1990. Pp. 101-120 in Women, Health, and Medicine: A Historical Handbook, R.D. Apple, ed. New York: Garland.

Brandt, A.M. 1985. Racism and research: The case of the Tuskegee Syphilis Study. In:Sickness and Health in America, 2nd ed., J.W. Leavitt and R.L. Number, eds. Madison: University of Wisconsin Press.

Cotton, D.J., He, W.L., Feinberg, J., and Finkelstein, D.M. 1993. Determinants of accrual of women to a large, multicenter HIV/AIDS clinical trials program in the United States. *Journal of Acquired Immune Deficiency* 6:1322-1328.

DeBruin, D.A. 1994. Justice and the inclusion of women in clinical studies: A conceptual framework. In: Women and Health Research: Ethical and Legal Issues of Including Women in Clinical Studies, Volume 2, A. Mastroianni, R. Faden, and D. Federman, eds. Washington, D.C.: National Academy Press.

Gamble, V.N., and Blustein, B.E. 1994. Racial differentials in medical care: Implications for research on women. In: Women and Health Research: Ethical and Legal Issues of Including Women in Clinical Studies, Volume 2, A. Mastroianni, R. Faden, and D. Federman, eds. Washington, D.C.: National Academy Press.

Gould, S.J. 1981. The Mismeasure of Man. New York: W.W. Norton & Company.

Hahn, R.A. 1992. The state of federal health statistics on racial and ethnic groups. *Journal of the American Medical Association* 267:268-271.

Healy, B. 1991. The Yentl syndrome. *New England Journal of Medicine* 324(4):274-276.

Hurh, W.M., and Kim, K.C. 1982. Methodological problems in the study of Korean immigrants: Conceptual, interactional, sampling and interviewer training difficulties. Pp. 81-93 in Methodological Problems in Minority Research, Occasional Paper No. 7, W.T. Liu, ed. Chicago: Pacific/Asian American Mental Health Research Center.

Jones, J.H. 1993. Bad Blood: The Tuskegee Syphilis Experiment, 2nd ed. New York: Free Press.

*Journal of the American Medical Association.* 1991. Special issue on Hispanic health. 265(2).

Krieger, N., and Bassett, M. 1986. The health of black folk: Disease, class, and ideology in science. *Monthly Review* 38:74-85.

Kuhn, T.S. 1970. The Structure of Scientific Revolutions, 2nd ed. Chicago: University of Chicago Press.

Lex, B.W., and Norris, J.R. 1994. Health Status of American Indian and Alaska native women.

Women and Health Research: Ethical and Legal Issues of Including Women in Clinical Studies, Volume 2, A. Mastroianni, R. Faden, and D. Federman, eds. Washington, D.C.: National Academy Press.

Mannheim, K. 1936. Ideology and Utopia: An Introduction to the Sociology of Knowledge. New York: Harcourt Brace Jovanovich.

Muldoon, M.F., Manuck, S.B., and Matthews, K.A. 1990. Lowering cholesterol concentrations and mortality: A quantitative review of primary prevention trials. *British Medical Journal* 301:309-314.

Nagel, E. 1961. The Structure of Science. New York: Harcourt, Brace and World.

NAS (National Academy of Sciences). 1989. On Being A Scientist. Washington, D.C.: National Academy Press.

Popper, K.R. 1981. The Logic of Scientific Discovery, 3rd ed. Boston: Routledge & Kegan Paul.

Presser, H. 1965. Sterilization and Fertility Decline in Puerto Rico, Population Monograph AE13. Berkeley: University of California Press.

Rodriguez-Trias, H. 1976. Women, health and law: Guidelines on sterilization under attack. *Women and Health* 1:30-31.

Schensul, S.L., Borrero, MG., Barrera, V., Backstrand, J., and Guarnaccia, P. 1982. A Model of fertility control in a Puerto Rican community. *Urban Anthropology* 1(1).

Scrimshaw, S.C., and Pasquariella, B. 1970. Obstacles to sterilization in one community. *Family Planning Perspectives* 2(4):40-42.

Sherwin, S. 1994. Women in clinical studies: A feminist view. Women and Health Research: Ethical and Legal Issues of Including Women in Clinical Studies, Volume 2, A. Mastroianni, R. Faden, and D. Federman, eds. Washington, D.C.: National Academy Press.

Sullivan, L.W. 1991. Effect of discrimination and racism on access to health care. *Journal of the American Medical Association* 266:2674.

Vasquez-Calzada, J.L. 1973. La esterilizacion femenina en Puerto Rico. *Revista de Ciencias Sociales* 17(3):281-308.

Wennberg, J.E. 1991. Unwanted variations in the rules of practice. *Journal of the American Medical Association* 265(10):1306-1307.

Williams, D.R. In press. Race in health services research: Past, present, and future. Health Services Research.

Williams, D.R., Lavizzo-Mourey, R., and Warren, R.C. 1993. Race in the health of America: Problems, issues, and directions. Submitted to *Public Health Reports.*

Wysowski, D.K., Kennedy, D.L., and Gross, T.P. 1990. Prescribed use of cholesterol-lowering drugs in the United States, 1978 through 1988. *Journal of the American Medical Association* 263(16):2185-2188.

Yu, E.S.H. 1994. Legal and ethical issues relating to the inclusion of Asian/Pacific Islanders in clinical studies. Women and Health Research: Ethical and Legal Issues of Including Women in Clinical Studies, Volume 2, A. Mastroianni, R. Faden, and D. Federman, eds. Washington, D.C.: National Academy Press.

Yu, E.S.H., and Liu, W.T. 1992. U.S. national health data on Asian Americans and Pacific Islanders: A research agenda for the 1990s. *American Journal of Public Health* 82(12):1645-1652.

Zambrana, R.E. 1994. The inclusion of Latino women in clinical and research studies: Scientific suggestions for assuring legal and ethical integrity. Women and Health Research: Ethical and Legal Issues of Including Women in Clinical Studies, Volume 2, A. Mastroianni, R. Faden, and D. Federman, eds. Washington, D.C.: National Academy Press.

# 6

# Legal Considerations

Legal considerations governing research on human subjects issue both from federal and state laws and from the institutional framework of sponsor agencies and research organizations that interpret and implement these laws. At the federal level, Congress has passed statutes and various federal agencies have promulgated regulations and guidelines to govern research on human subjects, including policies directly pertinent to the participation of women in clinical studies. The extent to which the individuals and organizations involved in the conduct of research must adhere to these policies depends on the type of policy: statutes and regulations must be followed by public and private entities, while guidelines are recommendations. Guidelines lack the force of law, but nevertheless have been quite effective in eliciting the desired behavior. Guidelines are also highly influential in setting standards for appropriate conduct.

The U.S. Constitution, with its protections of individual rights and provisions for equal protection under the law, provides further constraints on the behavior of public organizations and the private individuals and entities who work for them. Those involved in the conduct of human research also are governed by state constitutions, statutes, regulations, and liability decisions. Developed primarily through state appellate court decisions, the record of liability decisions is known as the *law of torts*. State tort liability rules are relevant to both the inclusion of women in, and the exclusion of women from, clinical studies. The greatest fears about liability for inclusion stem mainly from the possibility of injury to offspring resulting from women's participation in clinical drug trials.

## INSTITUTIONAL FRAMEWORK

Health-related research and development in the United States is supported by the federal government (predominantly through the National Institutes of Health [NIH]), the pharmaceutical industry, and private foundations. This institutional structure can affect the conduct of research because it is the source not only of funding, but also of procedures for reviewing the ethics of scientific research—including whether a proposed plan for selecting research participants is just—and of the legal requirements applicable to research.

NIH, located within the Public Health Service (PHS) of the Department of Health and Human Services (DHHS), is the single largest supporter of biomedical and behavioral research and development (health R&D) in the world. NIH underwrites approximately 73 percent of all health R&D supported by the U.S. federal government, and about 30 percent of all health R&D in the United States. In fiscal year 1992 the projected NIH health R&D budget was $8.4 billion (NIH, 1992).

NIH is an extraordinarily complex organization. It includes a federation of 16 institutes, the National Library of Medicine, two divisions, and four centers. All of these components are coordinated by the Office of the Director. NIH policies have a profound effect on other organizations that have health-related missions, including other federal agencies, awardee institutions, and private foundations and corporations that support or conduct health R&D. Many institutions simply adopt NIH policies and procedures. Other organizations, both public and private, adapt NIH policies to suit their own structures and needs.

Most NIH funding components have a twofold structure. Extramural programs support health R&D projects carried out by research institutions throughout the United States and in at least 80 nations worldwide. Intramural programs, operated by federal employees, conduct research on the NIH campus in Bethesda, Maryland, and at a number of other locations throughout the country (Maryland, North Carolina, Colorado, Florida, and other states). Approximately 88 percent of the NIH research budget is disbursed to nonfederal institutions through grants-in-aid, contracts, and cooperative agreements (NIH, 1992). Awards are made by NIH funding components operating with the advice of a large and carefully regulated peer review system. Grant applications submitted to NIH by extramural institutions are typically reviewed by initial review groups (IRGs), commonly called study sections, that conduct scientific merit review and assign a priority score to each application that it recommends for funding. Approximately 20 percent of applications recommended for funding are actually funded in any given fiscal year.

In addition to their responsibilities for assessing scientific merit, IRGs also are asked to identify ethical concerns associated with proposed research in relation to the rights and welfare of human research subjects, care and use of laboratory animals, and scientific misconduct. If an IRG or an NIH staff person raises an ethics concern, a bar to funding is entered into the computerized grant-tracking system. No award can be made in support of a barred project until and unless the concern has been resolved. Most grant applications also are reviewed by a national advisory council or board that considers program relevance and the public importance of the application. Boards and councils also have authority to raise ethical concerns that place a bar to funding. Ethics concerns raised by IRGs are reviewed and resolved by national advisory boards or councils.

Contract proposals and cooperative agreements for biomedical and behavioral research are reviewed in a manner similar to that utilized to review grant applications. Technical Evaluation Groups (TEGs) carry out assessment of the proposal in a manner analogous to that of IRGs. As is the case for IRGs, TEGs are expected to identify any ethics concerns associated with proposals for contracts or cooperative agreements. No contract or cooperative agreement can be finalized until and unless ethics concerns have been resolved.

In making awards, NIH and other PHS agencies operate under the general authority of the Public Health Service Act, which requires the secretary of DHHS to operate a wide variety of health-related regulatory, research, demonstration, and service programs. Responsibility for these programs is delegated by the secretary, or in some cases directly by the Congress, to the agencies and program directors throughout PHS.

Regulatory responsibility for protecting the rights and welfare of human research subjects has been delegated to the Office for Protection from Research Risks (OPRR). Although that office is located within NIH for organizational purposes, it acts on behalf of the secretary of DHHS. The primary instrument that OPRR uses in meeting its responsibility is the promulgation and implementation of regulations codified in the Code of Federal Regulations (C.F.R.) for the protection of human subjects. Those regulations require that, before awardee institutions are permitted to carry out research involving human subjects, they must provide adequate assurance to OPRR that they will comply with the regulations. The primary requirement of the regulations is that before work is begun and at intervals of no more than one year during the conduct of research involving human subjects, each research project shall be reviewed and approved by an institutional review board (IRB). The U.S. Food and Drug Administration (FDA) has also issued regulations at 21 C.F.R. 50 & 56 that include congruent requirements for IRB review of studies involving experimental drugs, devices, and biologics (see below).

IRBs are administrative bodies established to protect the rights and welfare of human research subjects recruited to participate in research activities conducted under the auspices of their affiliated institutions. Each IRB has authority to approve, require modifications in, or disapprove all research activities that fall within its jurisdiction.

The FDA, another PHS agency, functions under the Food, Drug and Cosmetic Act (FDCA). The FDCA provides the commissioner of FDA with authority and responsibility to regulate (among other articles) the testing and marketing of drugs, biologics, and medical devices involved in interstate commerce. The commissioner also is subject to policies and regulations issued by or under the authority of the secretary of DHHS and by many of the provisions of the PHS Act. In those rare instances when the FDA conducts clinical research, that research is subject to DHHS regulations. When NIH conducts or supports clinical studies involving the testing of investigational drugs, biologics, or devices, NIH and NIH awardee institutions are subject to FDA regulations governing such items. Institutions that conduct clinical studies funded by NIH or another PHS agency involving drugs, biologics, or medical devices are subject to all applicable policies and regulations of both NIH and FDA.

Institutions conducting research on drugs, biologics, and medical devices without any public funding, including research conducted by scientists in the employ of pharmaceutical companies and research conducted by academic scientists and others supported by the pharmaceutical industry or private foundations, are subject only to federal policies promulgated by FDA. According to the Pharmaceutical Manufacturers Association (PMA), the pharmaceutical industry contributes just over half of total health research dollars—$10.9 billion in 1992 (PMA, 1992). Industry research is carried out by pharmaceutical companies without federal funding either on-site or at universities. Privately funded pharmaceutical research carried out in a university setting, however, may be subject to DHHS regulations, because individual institutional policies frequently require investigators to conform to DHHS policy, independent of the funding source of a particular study. Private foundations (such as the Pew Foundation) and professional organizations (e.g., the American Lung Association) underwrite a much smaller, but not insignificant, percentage of health research. Such privately funded, nonpharmaceutical research would technically not be subject to any federal policies, but again, if conducted at an institution that receives federal funds, it would likely be subject to DHHS policy.

## CURRENT FEDERAL POLICIES

Current federal policies that affect equity in clinical studies take the form of statutes, regulations, and agency guidelines and memoranda. These policies govern research funded, conducted, or otherwise regulated by the federal government, its agencies, and departments. The policies vary: some appear to promote inclusion of both genders, others refer to inclusion of women and minorities, and still others specify conditions applicable to women of childbearing potential and pregnant women. Application of a particular policy may depend on funding origin (e.g., NIH, Department of Veterans Affairs, Department of the Army, private funding, and the like), type of research (e.g., drug development or observational study), nature of condition studied (e.g., life threatening), or fertility status of the proposed study participant (e.g., post-menopausal women, pregnant women, women of childbearing potential, men). Particularly in the area of drug development, clinical studies that receive federal funding or are performed at institutions supported by federal funding may be subject to a number of policies prior to a drug's entrance into the market. Recently such policies have become more consistent.

These sometimes overlapping policies are perhaps best understood through evaluation on an agency-by-agency basis. We will begin with a discussion of the policies of or affecting DHHS-funded research, focusing particularly on NIH and FDA policies. This will be followed by a discussion of relevant policies of other federal agencies and departments. Because many policies have been revised since 1990, the rationale for revising the earlier policy will be noted where relevant and available. In addition, the type of study, the condition studied, and any provisions to encourage the performance of scientific analyses to identify gender differences will be highlighted. Finally, where relevant, provisions applicable to fertile women will be contrasted with policies applicable to fertile men.

### National Institutes of Health

As of this writing, NIH policy on study population composition of intramural and extramural research is in transition. The future policy is reflected in Section 131 of the recent NIH reauthorization legislation, the National Institutes of Health Revitalization Act of 1993 (P.L. 103-43, 107 Stat. 133 to be codified at 42 U.S.C. 289a-2). This provision of the law mandates the inclusion of women and racial and ethnic groups in NIH intramural and extramural research. It is to be implemented in fiscal year 1995 through NIH guidelines scheduled to be published in December 1993; draft versions of these guidelines were not available to the committee.

The NIH policy on study population composition currently in effect is expected to be revised for implementation during the transition to the legis- latively mandated policy (J. LaRosa, deputy director of the NIH Office of Research on Women's Health, personal communication, October 1993). The policy in effect as of this writing was introduced in 1990 and consists of five components:

1.  the August 1, 1990, NIH policy memorandum on inclusion of women and minorities applicable to intramural research;
2.  the August 1990 policy notice entitled "NIH/ADAMHA Policy Con- cerning Inclusion of Women in Study Populations," applicable to extramu- ral research;
3.  the September 1990 policy notice entitled "NIH/ADAMHA Policy Concerning Inclusion of Minorities in Study Populations," applicable to extramural research;
4.  an explanatory memorandum entitled "NIH Instruction and Infor- mation Memorandum OER 90-5" describing the application of the two policy notices applicable to extramural research;
5.  the recently instituted requirements in PHS grant applications and continuation applications to identify proposed and recruited study popula- tions by gender and minority composition.

The legislative mandate and its implementing guidelines will likely super- sede at least the first four components of the current policy. It is possible that the PHS grant application will be modified as well, to accommodate the policy changes.

The current NIH policy, which became effective in February 1991 (re- ferred to collectively here as the "1991 NIH Policy") will only be briefly described, while the new legislative mandate (referred to here as the "Act") will be discussed in detail below, highlighting areas of known controversy.

## The 1991 NIH Policy

Following the issuance of the 1990 GAO report, NIH promulgated a strengthened policy to govern the awarding of federal research grants. The new policy applies to a wide variety of *extramural* clinical research projects, including:

> Human biomedical and behavioral studies of etiology, epidemiology, pre- vention (and preventive strategies), diagnosis, or treatment of diseases, disorders or conditions, including but not limited to clinical trials.

Standard language articulating the extramural policy now appears in all requests for proposals (RFPs) announced in the *NIH Guide for Grants and Contracts*:

Applications for grants and cooperative agreements that involve human subjects are required to include minorities and both genders in study populations so that the research findings can be of benefit to all persons at risk of the disease, disorder, or condition under study.

The applicant must describe the proposed study population composition and provide a "compelling" justification for gender or racial and ethnic group exclusion. The investigator must also address gender and racial and ethnic issues "in developing a research design and sample size appropriate for scientific objectives of the study." The *NIH Policy Notice* further explains that the inclusion of women and racial and ethnic groups in study populations will be considered a matter of scientific and technical merit in peer review.

What constitutes a "compelling" reason for exclusion has generated debate both within the scientific community and within Congress (Wittes and Wittes, 1993). The explanatory memorandum to NIH staff and peer advisory groups directs them to consider sufficient only "strong scientific or practical reasons" for the exclusion of women or racial and ethnic groups from clinical research. Some of the potentially "acceptable" justifications listed include: research on a "predominantly or exclusively a male condition" (e.g., prostate cancer); research that presents an "unacceptable risk for women of childbearing age"; certain pilot and feasibility studies in which "gender differences may not be germane"; research in an area that "has already been extensively studied in women"; and in certain instances, studies that would be "prohibitively expensive" (NIH, 1990).

Monitoring of study populations is accomplished through reporting requirements specified in PHS grant and continuation applications. These applications require awardees to identify annually proposed and actually enrolled study populations according to gender and the five designated racial and ethnic categories (American Indian/Alaskan Native, Asian/Pacific Islander, Black [not of Hispanic origin], Hispanic, and White [not of Hispanic origin]). A summary of study population composition during the first full year of the policy's implementation is expected to be issued by NIH soon.

Most of the NIH *intramural* research program is subject to a different, less restrictive policy that requires only that gender-based exclusions be indicated and a "clear rationale" be provided. It currently reads, in its entirety:

The inclusion of women must be considered in the study populations for all clinical research efforts. Exceptions would be studies of diseases which exclusively affect men or where involvement of pregnant women may expose the fetus to undue risks. Gender differences should be noted and evaluated. If women are not to be included, a clear rationale should be provided for their exclusion.

In order to provide more precise information to the medical community, it is recommended that publications resulting from NIH- or ADAMHA-conducted research specify, in the abstract or summary, the gender(s) of the research subjects or patients [Rall, 1990].

Large-scale intramural projects that are implemented through contracts are not subject to the foregoing policy, but rather are considered part of the extramural program for policy purposes.

*The Act* The NIH Revitalization Act of 1993 became law on June 10, 1993. The Act requires that women and ethnic and racial groups be included as subjects in each intramural and extramural clinical research project supported by NIH. It further requires that a *clinical trial* that includes women and racial and ethnic minorities as participants be designed and carried out to provide for valid analysis of whether the variables being studied affect these subpopulations differently than other participants. Furthermore, NIH is instructed to conduct or support outreach programs for recruitment and retention of women and racial and ethnic group participants in clinical research projects. The law allows for exemptions in cases of research that are inappropriate with respect to the health of the subjects, the purpose of the research, or other circumstances determined by NIH.

NIH is required to promulgate implementing guidelines by December 7, 1993. These guidelines are to specify when the inclusion of women and members of racial and ethnic groups as subjects in clinical research is inappropriate; how clinical trials must be designed to have adequate representation of subpopulations to distinguish whether a treatment affects a subpopulation differently than the other members of a research project; and the operation of outreach programs.

The Act includes express instructions for the NIH guidelines. For example, it specifically prohibits cost considerations as a reason for determining that the inclusion of women and racial and ethnic groups is inappropriate for a *clinical trial*. In *other clinical research projects*, however, an exception from the prohibition on cost considerations is allowed when the data that would be obtained by the research project is or will be obtained through other means that provide data of comparable quality. An example of where NIH may allow the exclusion of certain subpopulations on cost grounds is where a body of research on those groups exists and will be analyzed for differential response through other means, such as meta-analysis. Another exception from the prohibition of cost considerations involves cases where there is already a substantial body of scientific data demonstrating that there is no significant difference between subpopulations in the effects of the variable being studied. This prohibition on the consideration of cost differs from the 1991 NIH Policy, which allows cost to be an acceptable rationale for women's exclusion from certain clinical trials.

NIH has been provided with some degree of latitude in the development of their guidelines. For example, the act requires that clinical trials be designed and performed to enable a *valid analysis* of whether women or racial and ethnic groups respond differently than other subjects in the research. Concern has been expressed about the interpretation and implications of this clause. (IOM, 1993; Wittes and Wittes, 1993). The language of the report suggests the intent of Congress:

> Although the Committee has given the Director of NIH the general authority to define [valid analysis] . . . the Committee intends for that definition to include an analysis of not only whether differences among study populations exist statistically, but an analysis of what those differences are as well as their relative importance for various population subgroups in the study.

This would indicate that women and racial and ethnic groups are to be enrolled in clinical research projects in numbers large enough to provide statistical significance, and that the analysis of such research is to include distinctions among and between the various population groups, including women. These concerns have already been discussed in Chapter 4.

The NIH policy does not automatically require that study designs provide statistical power to perform gender analysis except "whenever there are scientific reasons to anticipate differences between men and women." Those who favor the language in the Act over that in the NIH policy contend that the scientific literature on gender-mediated effects is sufficiently sparse that one will not always be able to "anticipate" such differences (S. Wood, scientific director of the Congressional Caucus for Women's Issues, personal communication, May 1993).

Other provisions of the Act require NIH to establish internal and external committees to advise it on issues in women's health research, including gender differences in clinical drug trials and disease etiology, course, and treatment. The Act also requires NIH to determine the extent of women's representation as senior physicians and scientists in the institutes and to carry out activities to increase the extent of such representation. Finally, the Act mandates the creation of a national data system and clearinghouse on research for women's health (see Chapter 2).

The NIH Revitalization Act directs NIH to define the terms "minority group" and "subpopulations." The Act does not clarify the extent of required inclusion of racial and ethnic groups in clinical research projects. The reasons for the unequal legislative specificity between women and minority groups is discussed in the House Committee on Energy and Commerce report accompanying the bill: the committee explained that representative inclusion of minority groups poses a complex problem because not only are there variations between Caucasians and people of color, but there are also variations among variations (or subpopulations) of the same racial or ethnic group. The report emphasized the importance of identifying such variations in clinical studies, but explains that this statutory language was chosen to prevent quotas or numerical goals for participation in clinical research projects (U.S. Congress, 1993).

### Food and Drug Administration Policies

FDA policies concerning the inclusion of women in clinical studies are reflected in guidelines. It is important to note that guidelines do not have the force of law or regulation, and they do not have to go through the same public comment procedures as regulations. Guidelines are not binding on the agency, nor do they create or confer any rights, privileges, or benefits for or on any person. They are provided as an aid to organizations involved in the evaluation of new drugs for FDA approval who wish to market such drugs. FDA guidelines are used to specify the information that data reviewers of such applications will expect in the research that supports the safety and efficacy of a drug.

There are three FDA guidelines that are particularly relevant to inclusion of women in clinical trials. Two of these are discussed in detail; discussion of a 1988 guideline is incorporated into the discussion of the 1993 guideline, where its content has been reiterated.

### 1977 Guidelines

In 1977 the FDA issued guidelines for drug development: "General Considerations for the Clinical Evaluation of Drugs." The 1977 guidelines specifically stated that pregnant women and "women who are at risk of becoming pregnant" should be excluded from Phase I studies. They further recommended that a "woman of childbearing potential" be excluded from "large-scale clinical trials" (i.e., Phase III studies) until all three segments of the FDA Animal Reproduction Guidelines have been completed. The guidelines further provided that "if adequate information on efficacy and relative safety has been amassed during Phase II, women of childbearing potential may be included in further studies provided Segment II and the female part of Segment I of the animal reproductive studies have been completed" (FDA, 1977: 10). Segment I animal testing covers fertility and reproductive performance; Segment II covers teratogenesis; and Segment III covers perinatal and postnatal effects.

Women of childbearing potential, however, could receive investigational drugs in the absence of adequate animal reproduction studies when: (1) the drug was considered to be a life-saving or life-prolonging measure (e.g., cancer therapy), (2) the drug belonged to a class of compounds for which teratogenic potential had already been established in animals, or (3) the woman had been "institutionalized" for a period of time adequate to verify that she was not pregnant. When, under this exception, an investigational drug is used to treat a serious disease, the guidelines recommend that the investigator point out the lack of reproduction studies during the informed consent process, test the woman for pregnancy, and advise her of contraceptive measures. As Merton (1994) notes, the guidelines do not mandate the performance of reproduction studies at any time, and, further, do not mention how the results of such studies should affect the inclusion of women.

Lactating women are specifically mentioned in the guidelines, with the recommendation that excretion of the drug or its metabolites should be determined when feasible prior to their usage of the drug. If a woman becomes pregnant during the trial, the guidelines recommend fetal follow-up.

The guidelines broadly defined a woman of childbearing potential as a "premenopausal female capable of becoming pregnant" (FDA, 1977). Included in the definition were women on oral, injectable, or mechanical contraception; women who were "single"; and women whose partners had been vasectomized or were using mechanical contraception. This exclusion was based on a concern that women might become pregnant during the course of a clinical trial and a judgment that the potential risks of exposing a fetus to an experimental drug of unknown fetal toxicity were greater than the potential benefits of the information that would be gathered by including women of childbearing potential in these early trials.

Critics of the 1977 FDA guidelines had questioned for years whether the guidelines reflected gender stereotyping (e.g., female susceptibility and male invulnerability) more than concerns about good science (see Kinney et al., 1981). At a recent conference evaluating the issues concerning the inclusion of women in clinical trials, cosponsored by FDA and the Food and Drug Law Institute, critics claimed that an asymmetry existed in the risk-benefit analyses for research on men of reproductive potential and women of reproductive potential. They noted that according to the guidelines, research involving agents thought to cause reproductive harm in male animals could be conducted in men depending on "the nature of the abnormalities, the dosage at which they occurred, the disease being treated, the importance of the drug, and the duration of drug administration" (FDA, 1977). In practice this meant that even a drug known to have teratogenic effects in animals could be tested in men if they were simply informed of the risks and advised not to conceive while participating in the trial. The 1977 guidelines would have excluded women of reproductive potential from such trials based on the fact that potential offspring might be harmed.

The background paper accompanying recently issued FDA guidelines explains that the 1977 guidelines may have discouraged participation of women in drug development studies and may have resulted in a "paucity of information about the effects of drugs in women" (FDA, 1993: 4). As explained by FDA, the 1977 guidelines had come to be considered by many to be "rigid and paternalistic, leaving virtually no room for the exercise of judgment by responsible female research subjects, physician investigators, and IRBs" (FDA, 1993).

## 1993 Guideline

FDA released a new guideline, "Guideline for the Study and Evaluation of Gender Differences in the Clinical Evaluation of Drugs," on July 22, 1993. This guideline modifies and revises the section of the 1977 version concerning inclusion of women of childbearing potential in clinical trials. The introduction to this guideline indicates that the broad principles that are outlined for the inclusion of women in the early phases of clinical trials will also be applied to FDA approval processes for biological products and medical devices.

The new guidelines provide four underlying observations that persuaded the agency of the need for revision of the 1977 and 1988 directives on women in clinical drug trials. These observations are:

• Variations in response to drugs, including gender-related differences, can arise from pharmacokinetic (the effect of the body on the drug) differences or pharmacodynamic (the effect of the drug on the body) differences.

• Gender-related variations in drug effects may arise from a variety of sources (e.g., differences in biology, behavior, etc.) that can affect the pharmacokinetics of some drugs. Identification of these effects enhances the ability to treat both genders appropriately.

• In the evaluation of potential gender-related differences, evaluation of pharmacokinetic differences should precede pharmacodynamic differences because they are more common and because they can be used as an indicator of possible need for later pharmacodynamic studies that further narrow the affected variables for a drug.

• Since there are few documented gender-related pharmacodynamic differences of clinical significance, and pharmacodynamic/effectiveness studies may be difficult to conduct, such studies are not routinely necessary. However, pharmacokinetic studies and the development of blood concentration data to detect important pharmacodynamic and effectiveness differences related to gender are still needed.

*Inclusion of both genders in clinical studies* The guideline explains that subjects in a given clinical study should reflect the population that will receive the drug when it is marketed. Although the explicit exclusion of women from Phase I and early Phase II trials is lifted, the new guideline encourages but *does not* create a strict requirement that women be included in the early phases of drug trials. Rather, FDA now expects analysis of clinical data in drug applications to identify whether there is a gender difference in the response to the drug, and, if so, the basis of the gender difference (if it can be determined).

The guideline suggests that patients of both genders be included in the same trial to permit direct comparison of genders within the studies. The guideline also explicitly discredits routine exclusion of women from bioequivalence trials because changes during the menstrual cycle may cause intrasubject variability (differences or variations in an individual's response to the same amount of drug). Instead, inclusion of women in these studies is expected to indicate if there is a possible need for concern about the variations in response to a drug based on the hormonal fluctuations of the menstrual cycle.

*Analysis of effectiveness and adverse effects by gender*   This section reiterates FDA's 1988 guidelines for clinical and statistical sections of new drug applications, "Guideline for the Format and Content of the Clinical and Statistical Sections of New Drug Applications." The new guideline outlines FDA's expectations for the data analyses of gender differences and other subgroup differences, which are expected to be performed and explained in an application for approval of a new drug. Depending on the findings of these analyses, FDA may require further testing of a drug on specific populations to determine if there are instances in one or more populations where the drug is not as effective as in the overall population, or if there are instances of adverse reactions distinct to a certain population.

*Defining the pharmacokinetics of the drug in both genders*   FDA emphasizes the importance of pharmacokinetic studies and pharmacokinetic screens to define gender-related differences in drug responses. It recommends the use of "pilot studies" to ascertain the presence of significant pharmacokinetic differences *before* conducting controlled trials. This enables the early identification of possible variations in dosing regimens that can be built into the larger clinical trials. Emphasis is placed on the heightened importance of early pharmacokinetic studies for drugs with a narrow therapeutic range (drugs that have a small range of concentration between the point of effectiveness and the point of toxicity) where the generally smaller size of women could require modifications in dosing.

In addition, the FDA lists three gender-related facets of pharmacokinetics that "should be considered during drug development": (1) variations in pharmacokinetics caused by the menstrual cycle, including comparisons of premenopausal and postmenopausal patients as well as changes during the course of the menstrual cycle; (2) the effects on pharmacokinetics of estrogen replacement therapy and systemic contraceptives (oral contraceptives and long-acting progesterone such as Norplant®); and (3) the effect of oral contraceptives on pharmacokinetics.

*Gender-specific pharmacodynamic studies* Pharmacodynamic and effectiveness studies conducted separately on men and women are not expected by FDA unless the analyses by gender of clinical trials and pharmacokinetic screens indicate a significantly different gender-related response. In such cases, FDA will look for these additional studies. Once again, the importance of such additional studies increases should the early studies indicate a gender-related difference in response to a drug with a narrow therapeutic range.

*Precautions in clinical trials including women of childbearing potential* FDA will rely on the informed consent document and the investigator's brochure to advise participants of the need to take precautions to prevent the inadvertent exposure of a fetus to potentially toxic drugs. These documents should contain explanations of all available information about the degree of risk of fetal toxicity. It is FDA's belief that large-scale exposure of women of childbearing potential should not take place until after the results of animal toxicity tests are analyzed. It recommends that clinical protocols include provisions for the use of contraception (including counseling in the selection and use of contraception) or abstinence for the entire time a subject will be exposed to the drug (sometimes beyond the completion of the study), use of pregnancy tests before exposure to the drug, and timing studies in accordance with the menstrual cycle.

*Potential effects on fertility* In the clinical evaluation of drugs that carry the risk of causing abnormalities in reproductive organs or their function (as identified in animals), the risks of exposing individuals of reproductive potential must be weighed against the potential benefits of the drug. In cases where such drugs do proceed into clinical trials, such studies should include monitoring and laboratory studies, as well as long-term follow-up, to enable detection of potentially deleterious effects.

## Other DHHS Policies

### DHHS Policy on Pregnant Women as Research Subjects

In 1975, DHHS adopted regulations concerning pregnant women as research subjects. These regulations supplement the Model Federal Policy with respect to DHHS-funded research; the regulations have not been adopted by the other 15 federal agencies that adopted the Model Federal Policy. Selwitz and Wermeling (1992), however, have noted that the regulations have had an impact on IRB decision making at many research institutions, regardless of whether projects are funded by DHHS.

Subpart B of Part 46 of Title 45 of the Code of Federal Regulations is entitled "Additional Protections Pertaining to Research, Development, and Related Activities Involving Fetuses, Pregnant Women, and Human In Vitro Fertilization" and describes protections when the pregnant woman and/or the fetus is the subject of research. Where the pregnant woman is the subject of research, the regulations specify that research cannot be approved except where "appropriate" studies on animals and nonpregnant individuals have been performed (45 CFR section 46.206 (a)(2)) and

> (1) the purpose of the activity is to meet the health needs of the mother and the fetus will be placed at risk only to the minimum extent necessary to meet such needs, or (2) the risk to the fetus is minimal [45 CFR section 46.207 (a)]

"Minimal risk" is defined in another part of the regulations to mean that the probability and magnitude of harm or discomfort anticipated in the research are not greater than those ordinarily encountered in daily life, routine physical examinations, or psychological tests (45 CFR 46.102(i)).

In addition to the foregoing limitations, the regulations require that the "mother and father" be legally competent and give their informed consent after being fully informed regarding the possible impact of the research on the fetus. Exceptions are made for the father's informed consent if: the reason for the activity is to meet the health needs of the mother, his identity or whereabouts cannot reasonably be ascertained, he is not reasonably available, or the pregnancy resulted from rape (45 CFR sections 46.207(b)).

## Policies of Other Federal Agencies and Departments

The committee contacted the 15 other agencies and departments that have adopted the Model Federal Policy for Protection of Human Subjects (discussed above) to ask whether they had additional policies related to the inclusion of women in clinical studies. Two of those surveyed had such policies: the Department of the Army has a specific policy on pregnancy testing (Department of the Army, 1992), and the Department of Veterans Affairs has a policy generally promoting the inclusion of women in clinical studies (Department of Veterans Affairs, 1992). The Department of Energy explicitly recommends that the guidance provided in Subpart B of the DHHS regulations be followed if the proposed research involves pregnant women (Department of Energy, 1992).

## CONSTITUTIONAL ISSUES

All laws and policies of state and federal government are expected to conform to the ultimate source of legal authority in this country—the U.S. Constitution. The Fourteenth Amendment's express protections against laws that deny "equal protection" and "life, liberty, and property" are particularly relevant to questions of participation in clinical research. The Fourteenth Amendment, and the Bill of Rights generally, have been interpreted by the Supreme Court to require equal access to government health benefits, along with a high degree of personal liberty in matters affecting health care. This has led some legal experts and advocates to conclude that exclusion of women from government-sponsored or government-regulated research violates constitutional standards of liberty and equality.

Officials of federal agencies understand that their policies and activities may be subject to constitutional challenge and review. For example, a lawsuit seeking to invalidate a federal biomedical research policy would likely name as defendants the Department of Health and Human Services and its secretary. Private firms, such as pharmaceutical manufacturers, generally are not considered arms of the government. Nevertheless, a citizen's petition filed with the FDA in December 1992 argued that the policies and practices of the industry could count as government action, for purposes of construing the Fourteenth Amendment, to the extent that the FDA or other federal agencies encourage the firms that they closely regulate to exclude women from studies (NOW Legal Defense and Education Fund, 1992). Were industry action held to be government action, Fourteenth Amendment principles would apply to industry policies of exclusion.

### Liberty, Privacy, and Bodily Self-Determination

The Fourteenth Amendment provides that "No state shall . . . deprive any person of life, liberty, or property." This protection of bodily self-determination and private decisionmaking about matters closely affecting health is often labeled the "right to privacy." Women and their advocates have sometimes appealed to this right to protest exclusion from, for example, acquired immune deficiency syndrome (AIDS) research: women with AIDS or human immunodeficiency virus (HIV) infection have a right to choose for themselves whether to take on the health risks of drug research. Advocates say that the principles of private choice and good science should determine the extent of female participation in research, not the principle of government paternalism.

The Supreme Court has repeatedly held that decisional privacy about matters affecting health care is among the liberties protected by the Fourteenth Amendment. The Court has upheld this right with regard to the termination of artificial nutrition and hydration (*Cruzan v. Director, Missouri Department of Health*) and abortion (*Roe v. Wade*). The Court reaffirmed the right to private abortion decisionmaking in *Planned Parenthood of Southeastern Pennsylvania v. Casey*, in which it recognized the right of a woman "to choose to have an abortion before viability and to obtain it without undue interference from the State." While acknowledging a state interest in the life of at least some fetuses, the Court also stressed the importance of reproductive privacy for women's liberty, linking a woman's "unique" reproductive liberty to her ability "to participate equally in the economic and social life of the nation."

Unresolved for now is the question of the standard of review that the Court should apply in Fourteenth Amendment privacy cases relating to women's health. In *Roe v. Wade*, the Court applied a standard it calls "strict scrutiny." Under this standard, the Court strikes down laws or policies that constrain "fundamental" rights and liberties unless the government can cite a "compelling state interest" that cannot be furthered by "less restrictive means." In the *Cruzan* case, however, the Court applied a weaker standard of review known as "rational basis," under which the Court upholds laws or policies that are rationally related to a "legitimate state interest." A third standard of review appears to have been utilized in the *Casey* decision, where the Court considered whether the state laws in question "unduly burdened" the woman's Fourteenth Amendment right of private abortion decisionmaking. *Casey* did not expressly appeal to the idea of a general, "fundamental" right to privacy requiring "strict scrutiny" as *Roe v. Wade* had two decades earlier. As a consequence, there is uncertainty among lawyers and jurists about precisely what standard of review would apply in future Fourteenth Amendment privacy cases affecting women's health, including cases involving exclusion from research.

The uncertain status of privacy jurisprudence makes it difficult to predict the outcome of challenges to policies that exclude women from health research. Nevertheless, scholars have argued that *Cruzan's* recognition of a right to refuse artificial nutrition and hydration, premised on freedom from intervention in private decisionmaking related to health care, also implies a right to take part in risky clinical studies, i.e., if one can terminate one's own life, one should be able to assume the risk of taking an untested drug. This argument may be particularly strong when made on behalf of women suffering from terminal illnesses who seek access to experimental drug therapies.

## Privacy vs. Fetal Protection

Objections to women's participation in clinical studies are often premised on an interest in doing what is best for women's own health and well-being; but in some instances they are also based on an interest in fetal and child welfare. The former objection assumes that policy makers ought to protect women (but need not protect men to the same degree) from risky activities. The "right to refuse treatment" analogy rejects such intervention as unwarranted paternalism, suggesting instead that decisions affecting one's own physical person must be treated as personal and private. Objections based on fetal and child welfare assume that policymakers are entitled to limit women's choices where those choices impose risks on the unborn. If women have a constitutional right to abortion that is virtually unfettered in the early weeks of pregnancy, however, the case for fetal protection seems weak. Some have argued that the case for fetal protection is stronger if it is the children those fetuses will become (in pregnancies intended to go to term) that the policy seeks to protect (see, for example, Robertson, 1994; Steinbock, 1994).

Tribe (1991) and other constitutional experts assert that the unborn are not persons within the meaning of the Constitution, and that the case for fetal protection is without significant support. Yet the question of the legal status of the unborn is complex. The unborn are ascribed numerous legal interests, including those provided by the laws of inheritance and personal injury. *Casey* expressly recognizes a governmental interest in the welfare of an unborn fetus that "may become a child." Nevertheless, the Supreme Court has held to the principle that government may not deny women and their physicians the liberty to abort previable fetuses. Thus, both *Roe* and *Casey* are inconsistent with any notion that the previable fetus is a constitutional person with a right to life equivalent to that of newborns and children. *Casey* also invalidated provisions of a Pennsylvania statute requiring that pregnant women attest to having notified their spouses of plans to abort.[2] The Court saw no legally enforceable role for third-party notification and consent in the procreative decisionmaking of adult pregnant women. This is the strongest constitutional basis for an argument that husbands and fathers also have no legally enforceable role in deciding whether a pregnant woman may expose herself and a fetus to research-related health risks, even in the therapeutic context.

Some states have attempted to control the behavior of pregnant women in order to protect fetuses. Between 1982 and 1987, institutions in 18 states noted 36 different attempts to override maternal refusals of medical treatment, such as forced caesarean sections and intrauterine transfusions; judges issued court orders for an overwhelming majority (86 percent) of these interventions (Green, 1993).[3] Many states have also tried to prosecute women for engaging in behavior during pregnancy that is suspected or known to be risky for the fetus. For the most part, efforts to charge a pregnant woman with crimes ranging from delivering drugs to a minor and criminal abuse and neglect to disobeying doctor's orders have been unsuccessful. Courts have shown a reluctance to include a fetus in the definition of child in existing child abuse laws (Green, 1993). But where courts have been hesitant, state legislatures have not: 12 states have made it a crime for a pregnant woman to use drugs and alcohol, and 19 states have passed laws allowing prosecutors to charge women with child abuse if they give birth to children with illegal drugs in their blood (Green, 1993).

Since the Supreme Court has not ruled on the constitutionality of these state statutes and court decisions, the committee cannot draw any firm conclusions about whether fetal interests limit women's rights to decisional privacy. Until these fetal protectionist policies are challenged, they remain enforceable as law. As a result, equal protection rather than privacy principles may ultimately be a stronger basis for a constitutional test of policies that, on their face or in effect, exclude women from full participation in clinical research.

## Equal Protection

The wholesale exclusion of women from research would raise obvious equal protection concerns. So, too, would what constitutional lawyers term the "underinclusion" and "overinclusion" of women relative to men in clinical research. "Underinclusion" in this context could signify, for example, the inclusion of women in clinical research in numbers lower than good science requires; by contrast, "overinclusion" in this context could refer to the preferential inclusion of women in numbers great enough to diminish the scientific merit of the research.

The equal protection clause of the Fourteenth Amendment provides that: "No State shall . . . deny to any person within its jurisdiction the equal protection of the laws." Although this clause makes express reference only to "State" government, the Supreme Court has long held that it applies to both the state and federal government. Courts have recognized that the principle of equal protection is embodied also in other key provisions of the Constitution, including Article I and the due process clauses of the Fifth and Fourteenth Amendments. Significantly, each state has a constitution, and many state constitutions contain provisions similar to those found in the federal constitution that are held to require equal protection of the law.

The equal protection clause prohibits the federal government—including its regulatory agencies and research units—from engaging in certain forms of discriminatory disparate treatment. The Supreme Court has yet to decide a challenge to a demographic restriction on access to clinical studies, but legal experts maintain that research policies that result in the exclusion of women as a class, whether *on their face* (with explicit exclusionary language) or *in effect* (because they result in disproportionate participation of men and women), may be found to contradict the equal protection clause (Charo, 1994; Merton, 1992). Policies that explicitly favor participation of women in research also raise equal protection concerns.

The most controversial research policies have excluded women or categories of women through explicit policy language. For example, the 1977 FDA guidelines (now superseded) recommended the exclusion of women of childbearing potential from early phase drug trials; the regulations governing research on human subjects require that IRBs approve research on pregnant women only if it involves treatment for the mother or fetus and minimal risk to the fetus (45 C.F.R. § 46.207). Other policies, however, may exclude women because their aggregate effect is the "underinclusion" or exclusion of women from full participation in research. For example, if evidence is found that the benefits of participating in research accrue disproportionately to men, it could be argued that the federal research policies effectively result in disparate treatment of men and women. At the same time, it is conceivable that a man could challenge the constitutionality of the NIH Revitalization Act of 1993 if its language was legally determined to be an express preference for the participation of women in clinical studies and sufficient evidence was available to prove that the benefits of participation accrued disproportionately to men.

The Supreme Court has concluded that the equal protection clause restricts the right of the government to treat similarly situated persons and groups differently. Nevertheless, the Constitution does permit differential treatment that is, in the language of the federal courts, "reasonable"—that is, if government can cite a "rational basis" for discrimination that is tied to "legitimate state interests." A long-standing exception to this principle is the rule that merely reasonable disparate treatment premised on racial categories is presumptively unconstitutional. Legal restrictions that curtail the rights of any racial group are immediately suspect, and courts are required to subject such restrictions to its most rigid review standard: "strict scrutiny." Only in rare instances, when government can identify "compelling" state interests that can be promoted only by racial discrimination, will the courts permit a racial restriction to stand.

Today, legal restrictions that impair the equal treatment of women are also inherently suspect. As explained by Tribe (1987), "until the early 1970s, the Supreme Court routinely upheld sexually discriminatory laws whenever they could be rationally related to government purposes reflecting traditional views of the 'proper' relationship between men and women in American society." In the late 1970s, the Supreme Court held in *Craig v. Boren* that policies and practices involving gender classifications are constitutionally suspect. Establishing an "intermediate" level of scrutiny for gender discrimination cases, the Court held that gender classifications must have an "exceedingly persuasive justification" and be substantially related to "important governmental objectives."

Under this standard, women's treatment in the context of government research may be unconstitutional under the principle of equal protection if it results in disparate public benefits, unless there is an exceedingly persuasive justification. If a policy does not exclude women on its face, but its effect (alone or in combination with other policies) is a disproportionate accrual of benefits to men over women, a claim can theoretically be made that such a policy is unconstitutional under the equal protection clause. To successfully claim that a facially neutral policy results in discriminatory treatment in effect, however, the Court must find that the government agency or state actor implementing such a policy had the actual *intent* to discriminate (*Personnel Administrator of Massachusetts v. Feeney*). Unless intent can be shown, facially neutral policies that result in disparate impact need only show a rational relationship to a legitimate government objective. Under this level of scrutiny, the Court usually gives great deference to the government agency and upholds the policy.

## Policies That Exclude Pregnant Women

The federal regulation barring the use of pregnant women in research except in limited circumstances (45 C.F.R. § 46.207) is an example of a facially neutral policy (it can be classified as gender-neutral because it doesn't explicitly exclude *all women* as a class) that arguably results in disparate treatment of women (because only women can be pregnant). In a constitutional challenge to the regulation, the government would likely argue that the policy is linked to an important government objective—that of protecting potential life—and that there was no intent to discriminate against women in creating the pregnancy classification.

The question of whether the differential treatment of pregnancy represents a suspect gender classification was first dealt with in *Geduldig v. Aiello*. The Supreme Court held that the equal protection clause was not violated by California when it excluded pregnancy-related disability from coverage under the state's disability insurance program. The Court found that the classification in California's program was not between men and women but between pregnant and nonpregnant persons; despite the argument that only women can be pregnant, the Court found that this policy was not on its face treating women differently. Consequently, the Court construed the arguments of the plaintiffs to be an *in effect* challenge and inquired as to whether California intended to discriminate against women in designing the program. Finding no intent to discriminate, the Court then cited the state's "legitimate interest in maintaining a self-supporting . . . insurance program" and upheld the constitutionality of the program. This decision, permitting disparate treatment of pregnancy, appears to be directly relevant to any inquiry about the constitutionality of federal regulations governing research on pregnant women.

A more recent Supreme Court decision—*International Union, UAW v. Johnson Controls*—has sent a different signal about disparate treatment of pregnant women. Johnson Controls excluded pregnant and fertile women employees from selected jobs in its battery manufacturing plant out of concern about the effects of exposure to certain chemicals on the unborn and about its liability for injury to the fetus. Employees filed a lawsuit under Title VII of the Civil Rights Act of 1964, as modified by the Pregnancy Discrimination Act. Title VII prohibits sex-based employment discrimination, and the Pregnancy Discrimination Act makes it clear that for the purposes of Title VII, discrimination based on pregnancy is discrimination based on sex (*Newport News Shipping & Dry Dock Co. v. EEOC*). The Court held in favor of the employees, stating that women could give their informed consent to potentially risky employment and that Title VII did not permit the company to single out women in its concern about offspring.

*Johnson Controls* was brought under a federal civil rights statute governing private sector discrimination in the terms and conditions of employment, but the notion that it is wrongfully discriminatory to exclude women from a benefit on grounds of fetal protection could apply by analogy to the context of clinical studies. The employment-related finding in *Johnson Controls* may apply more directly to the research study context only in what Merton (1992) describes as the "rare circumstance that subjects are paid and their participation in research is fairly characterized as employment."

## Exclusion of Women of Childbearing Potential

Although the 1977 FDA guidelines that recommended the exclusion of women of childbearing potential have been superseded, there may be some value in analyzing the constitutionality of such a broad restriction under the equal protection clause. Categorical exclusion of *all* women of childbearing potential—without regard to an individual woman's actual childbearing capacities and intentions, or to the effect of the substance under study on the unborn—would arguably be unconstitutionally broad under the equal protection clause. Similarly, it can be argued that such policies are unconstitutionally underinclusive where they exclude only *women* of childbearing potential, ignoring fertile men whose reproductive capacities and offspring may be affected by the substance under study (see Chapter 7). Again, any policy that restricts the research participation of women of childbearing potential will also be questionable under the decision in *Johnson Controls*, in which the Court struck down an exclusion policy that applied to fertile women as well as to pregnant women.

## Policies That Favor Inclusion of Women

Equal protection challenges also apply to benign classifications, which favor treatment of one group over another, usually to remedy past discrimination. Affirmative action policies are examples of benign classifications. It could thus be argued that the NIH Revitalization Act, which calls for affirmative inclusion of women in clinical studies, could arguably be considered a benign classification. If the constitutionality of this statute is challenged by a man on grounds of disparate treatment, the intermediate scrutiny test developed in *Craig v. Boren* for application to exclusion would also be applicable to favored inclusion. The success of such a challenge would likely hinge on whether the government could present evidence of past discrimination against women in research to justify the disparate treatment.[4] The committee declines to speculate on the outcome of such a challenge, especially in light of currently available data on the participation of women (see Chapter 2).

## LIABILITY

Both individuals and organizations involved in the conduct of research must deal with another set of legal considerations—liability. Fear of potential legal liability has been cited as one of the chief reasons that some women have been excluded from clinical research (NAS, 1991; Flannery and Greenberg, 1994; Merton, 1992). The possibility of injuries to the women themselves, however, has not been the basis for this concern. Increasing the number of women in clinical studies will simply add them to the class of all clinical research participants, and concern about participant injuries has never been great enough to halt research involving human subjects. Rather, the focus of liability concerns is on possible injury to offspring when pregnant women and women of childbearing potential are included in clinical drug trials. Although recent evidence may indicate that exposure of the father to some chemicals may cause harm to a developing fetus (see Chapter 7), the focus has overwhelmingly been on the potential for harm to offspring resulting from the mother's exposure either before or after conception.

More recently, pharmaceutical companies have begun to recognize that they could also be liable for *not* including women in clinical research (Bush, 1993). For example, a pharmaceutical company may be liable if a drug that has never been tested in women is nevertheless marketed for use by both genders and prescribed for a woman who then suffers an adverse reaction. Similar approaches to liability could be used as well where men, or subpopulations of women or men, were not included in a study population but suffered an injury. This creates a paradox for pharmaceutical manufacturers whose efforts to exclude women in order to protect themselves from liability may actually risk liability for exclusion.

## Potential Liability for Inclusion

The threat of liability exists for injury to any subject of clinical research. Although fear of liability has never operated to exclude men as a class from participating in research, a general discussion of liability for research injuries is instructive in understanding how this liability operates in the context of research involving pregnant women and women of childbearing potential. The following sections discuss the incidence of research injuries, the legal theories that could serve as the basis for legal action, and the individuals and entities that might be found liable.

## Incidence of Research Injuries and Subsequent Legal Actions

The *reported* incidence of research injuries generally appears to be quite low. NIH and FDA do not require investigators or sponsors to report research injuries, and there is no registry of injuries for publicly or privately sponsored research. A 1975 survey of principal investigators found that only 3.7 percent of research participants had been injured, with less than 1 percent of the injured participants suffering permanently disabling or fatal injuries (Cardon et al., 1976). The incidence of injury in this survey was not separated by gender or by age; thus the incidence of injury to women, or to offspring as a result of women's participation in clinical studies, has not been quantified.

Legal recourse is sought in only a small percentage of research injuries, and an even smaller number ever reach court. The NIH Office of the General Counsel is only aware of three legal actions for clinical research injuries where NIH was involved in the past 20 years.[5] According to the FDA Office of the General Counsel, that agency has never been the subject of a legal action resulting from a clinical trial injury (R. Blumberg, personal communication, August 1993).

There have been approximately two dozen *reported* legal cases concerning research injuries—that is, cases in which a written opinion was officially published and thus available to courts, lawyers, and the public. Opinions are normally published in case reporters; occasionally, an opinion may be available only through on-line legal databases such as LEXIS and WESTLAW. For the most part, reported opinions are rendered by appellate courts and federal district courts. Cases that are decided at the state trial level usually are not reported, nor are injury claims that are settled out of court (case records are often sealed as part of the settlement agreement). Thus, the small number of reported research injury cases do not reflect all actions initiated as a result of research injury.

At a recent Institute of Medicine (IOM) workshop on AIDS vaccine clinical trials, the general counsel for a small U.S. pharmaceutical company stated that nine legal actions had been filed against his firm seeking damages for adverse reactions resulting from clinical trials of one drug. As of 1991 (the date of the workshop), the company had not lost a court judgment for any of these cases, but several cases had been settled at substantial cost to the company (IOM, 1991b).

Because of the extensive disclosure involved in the informed consent process, those injured in research seldom have a basis to pursue legal action (Flannery and Greenberg, 1994). When participants take part in the informed consent process, they may feel they have assumed the risks involved in research and therefore be less likely to initiate legal action (Clayton, 1994). Participants may also be less likely to start legal proceedings because they usually receive excellent medical care if they have an adverse reaction. In addition, corporations generally take action to avoid risk, and plaintiffs have difficulty in proving that their injuries were caused by the research. All of these considerations may contribute to the lack of legal activity in the area. With regard to injuries to offspring, until very recently FDA guidelines discouraged the use of women of childbearing potential in early phases of research; hence the full potential for liability for injuries to offspring may be unrealized.

Even though there are few reported cases of research-related injury, fear of liability has played a key role in the exclusion of women in their childbearing years and pregnant women from many clinical studies. Factors that contribute to the intimidating legal landscape include the following:

- Legal actions can be extremely costly to defend, even if the plaintiff's case is weak and the question of liability is uncertain, and companies are inclined to take any action that appears likely to eliminate or reduce the risk of becoming involved in litigation (Flannery and Greenberg, 1994)[6];
- variation in liability rules among the states;
- uncertainty introduced by having highly technical and complex scientific issues evaluated by a judge and jury untrained in the sciences;[7]
- a manufacturer's inability to rely on FDA approval as protection against liability;
- perception that the number of legal actions filed and the size of awards have increased dramatically in recent years;
- fear of loss of public confidence because of adverse publicity (IOM, 1990).

## Theories of Liability for Inclusion

Because of the paucity of reported decisions related to research-related injury, prediction of the risk of liability from the inclusion of women in clinical studies is difficult. Because of this difficulty, the committee found it helpful to examine the theories on which such an action might be brought. Legal actions for research injuries have generally been based in tort law, the branch of the law that allows persons injured by certain conduct to seek monetary compensation. Tort law is the province of state law, created through state legislation and the state "common law" developed through judicial decisions. Although variations exist among the states, state tort rules are similar enough that generalized statements of liability can be made. For example, many states, through their courts and state legislatures, have adopted portions of the *Restatement (Second) of Torts,* the American Law Institute's synthesis of the major principles of contemporary tort law (ALI, 1977). The three legal bases for a legal action for research injury are battery, negligence, and strict liability. The most common application of negligence in the area of research injury is lack of informed consent.

*Battery*   Battery generally is defined as unlawful and intentional bodily contact, directed at another person without that person's consent (Keeton et al., 1984). Battery is an *intentional* tort; thus an intentional contact that is unpermitted, harmful, or offensive is a necessary element. In the context of research, if someone is used as a research subject without his or her knowledge or consent, all of the potential defendants may face a legal action for battery. Damages awarded in a battery action will generally include *compensatory damages*, which are designed to compensate the plaintiff for any harm resulting from the contact and will include payment for medical expenses, loss of wages, and pain and suffering. *Punitive damages*, which are intended to punish the defendant for willful, injurious behavior, may also be awarded in a battery action (Keeton et al., 1984).

*Negligence*   Negligence is deviation from acceptable standards of conduct. To establish negligence, the plaintiff must prove that: (1) the defendant had a legal duty to the plaintiff; (2) the defendant breached that duty; (3) the plaintiff suffered an injury; and (4) this injury was caused by the defendant's breach of its duty (Keeton et al., 1984). The duty owed may be the general obligation that persons have to exercise reasonable care toward other people and their property. A duty may be mandated or implied by a statute, regulation, or guideline, as is the case in the context of research on human subjects. The duty also may be shaped by whether the defendant reasonably could have foreseen the injury to the plaintiff.

The existence of a duty will in turn create responsibilities on the part of the defendant to exercise due care. The level of care that a defendant must exercise to avoid liability, called the *standard of care,* is determined by what is reasonable under the circumstances. The defendant will be found to have breached a duty if his or her behavior fell below the standard of care (Keeton et al., 1984). In the research context, the standard of care is shaped in part by the conduct deemed reasonable when one is entrusted with human lives. Federal policies for research on human subjects also may help set the standard of care.

To recover damages for negligence, the plaintiff must also prove that the defendant's actions caused the injury. Causation can be a difficult concept: the plaintiff must show that, "but for" the actions of the defendant, the injury would not have occurred. This is "cause in fact." But the plaintiff must also establish legal cause, or proximate cause. The defendant is only responsible for the damages that are a *foreseeable* consequence of his or her behavior. For example, courts have differed as to whether a party may be liable for injuries to offspring that occur as a result of an injury to the woman before the child's conception (see below for more on preconception liability).

In most negligence cases, only compensatory damages are awarded. In cases where the defendant's behavior was reckless or an extreme departure from the standard of care, commonly known as gross negligence, however, some states allow a plaintiff to recover punitive damages as well (Keeton et al., 1984). Third parties may also recover money damages for injury to a research participant caused by negligence. For example, a spouse or child may claim loss of consortium, the legal term for the loss of "the society and affection" of the injured person.

Finally, while it is necessary that there be some injury in order to recover damages, the injury need not necessarily be tangible. In some cases, for example, plaintiffs exposed to toxic substances recovered damages for anxiety caused by fear of getting cancer (Reisman, 1992).

*Strict liability*    Pharmaceutical manufacturers, because they are in the business of selling a product, may also be held to the legal principles governing product liability. Under strict liability, a person injured by a product can recover damages without having to show that the manufacturer was negligent (ALI, 1977). Strict liability proponents believe that manufacturers should bear this cost because they can distribute the costs of injuries to all persons who benefit from the product through their power to set the market price of the product (Campbell, 1969).

A manufacturer may be strictly liable if it sells a product "in a defective condition unreasonably dangerous to the user or consumer" (ALI, 1977). A manufacturer may keep its product from being considered "unreasonably dangerous" by giving appropriate warnings; the adequacy of these warnings is often the legal issue in contention. In a research context, the manufacturer is not selling the drug directly to the participant; nevertheless, one state court rejected the notion that strict liability would not apply to drugs in the experimental phase because they were not sold (Merton, 1992, citing *Gaston v. Hunter*).

Courts in some states have exempted drug manufacturers from strict liability by adopting an explanatory comment from the *Restatement of Torts*. Comment k states that a drug is not unreasonably dangerous, and thus its manufacturer is not subject to strict liability, if the drug is "properly prepared and marketed and a proper warning is given" (ALI, 1977). Commentators have argued that drugs in the experimental phase are particularly strong candidates for "comment k protection," because the language of comment k specifically refers to experimental drugs: "new or experimental drugs as to which, because of lack of time and opportunity for sufficient medical experience, there can be no assurance of safety" (Flannery and Greenberg, 1994). States differ in the extent of their adoption of comment k for drugs; some states have chosen to apply its protection only on a case-by-case basis.

Some courts have found that manufacturers have a duty to warn consumers directly—for example, for prescription contraceptives (Flannery and Greenberg, 1994). Under the "learned intermediary doctrine," however, manufacturers can usually satisfy their duty to warn for prescription and investigational drugs by informing physicians and investigators of any risks of harm. The physicians are then responsible for prescribing drugs only for appropriate indications and for monitoring their use.

## Informed Consent

Legal actions for research injury based on a negligence theory frequently involve the doctrine of informed consent. Because nearly all research is conducted after securing consent from participants, most legal actions by participants for research injuries will be based on whether the information given to the participant before securing consent adequately warned of the potential risks (Reisman, 1992). The doctrine of informed consent requires that physicians secure consent from the patient before medical treatment is administered, and this consent must be based on information given to the patient about the risks and benefits of the proposed procedure and the alternatives (Wadlington, 1984).

There is a distinction between the nature of the consent necessary to avoid a legal action for battery and that necessary to avoid an action for negligence. Consent to avoid a charge of battery is a form of first-order assent to a bodily intervention, sometimes referred to as *simple consent*. By contrast, consent to avoid an action for negligence generally requires what has come to be called *informed consent,* a consent based on the disclosure of all facts "which are necessary to form the basis of an intelligent consent by the patient to the proposed treatment" (*Salgo v. Leland Stanford Jr. University*). In the context of research, if persons are subjected to a study without their knowledge or consent, any of the potential defendants may be sued for battery (see Appendix D). If the initial consent to participate has been secured but it was obtained without adequate disclosure of risks and alternatives, the legal action will be based on lack of informed consent, which is considered to be negligence.

This distinction is important. Damage awards for negligence will be smaller than those for battery, because they only compensate the plaintiff for his or her injuries; for an intentional tort such as battery, punitive damages may also be awarded. The statute of limitations—which limits the number of years during which a legal action can be initiated—is usually longer for a negligence action. For a battery, the plaintiff needs to prove there was an intentional contact with her body without her consent. In a negligence action for lack of informed consent, the patient will usually present the testimony of experts on how much information would be considered to be a reasonable disclosure under the circumstances. This is part of demonstrating to the court the standard of care for informed consent, which is necessary in order to prove that the defendant breached this standard. The plaintiff also must then prove that she would not have chosen to be a participant in the research had she been given more complete information (*Shack v. Holland*).

The federal regulations on informed consent for research will influence the standard against which a defendant will be judged; that is, whether the degree of disclosure was reasonable given the circumstances. Meeting these regulations, however, does not shield potential defendants from liability. The mechanisms for securing informed consent in any research protocol will also be subjected to scrutiny under the particular state's criteria for the standard of care for negligence actions. Some states allow physicians to set the standard by inquiring into the extent of disclosure that is customary for physicians practicing in the community. Other states apply a more objective standard: what a prudent person in the patient's position would want to know about the possible risks (Wadlington, 1984). Many states have adopted a more subjective standard based on how much information is needed in order to allow a particular patient (the plaintiff) to make a decision (Keeton et al., 1984).

A recent decision from a North Carolina court indicates that courts may require a higher standard for informed consent in nontherapeutic research injury cases. In *Whitlock v. Duke University*, the plaintiff, a participant in a nontherapeutic study looking at high-pressure nervous syndrome in underwater diving, signed a consent form advising him of known physical risks and the possibility of unknown risks. The plaintiff claimed he suffered organic brain damage from the dive and sued the researcher and the university, citing negligent failure to warn about the danger of brain damage. The court cited the DHHS regulations on informed consent for nontherapeutic research and held that the researcher and the university had a duty to inform the plaintiff of all "reasonably foreseeable" risks. Although the court found that in this particular case the risk of brain damage was not reasonably foreseeable, it nevertheless articulated a strict standard for informed consent to nontherapeutic research (Kobasic, 1988, citing *Whitlock*).

## Liability of Potential Defendants

Targets of legal action—potential defendants—in the research context may include public and private entities who sponsor or oversee research (such as NIH, FDA, and pharmaceutical manufacturing firms), as well as those who approve and conduct research (such as IRBs, investigators, physicians, and research institutions). If an offspring is injured as a result of a parent's participation in a drug trial, the parent could also be a defendant, together with the research sponsor (see below).

*Government agencies* The liability of government agencies, because they conduct research in the name of the federal government, is a special one and is spelled out in federal law. Historically, under the doctrine of sovereign immunity, the United States could not be sued, nor could its agencies and departments. The Federal Tort Claims Act (FTCA), passed in 1964, sharply restricted federal sovereign immunity; government agencies that conduct, sponsor, or oversee research, such as NIH and FDA, may now be held liable if a research participant is injured as a result of negligence (28 U.S.C. §§ 1346(b), 2674 [1964]). Plaintiffs must sue the government agency in order to recover; the Federal Employees Liability Reform and Tort Compensation Act of 1988 (P.L. 15-11) protects federal employees from personal liability for tortious actions committed within the scope of their employment. The federal government cannot be sued for injuries resulting from the negligence of persons not directly employed by the federal government but who are working with full or partial federal financial support. For example, NIH could not be sued for the negligence of an investigator in an extramural research protocol (*United States v. Orleans*).

FTCA prohibits legal actions for battery and those arising out of the exercise of a "discretionary function," a provision that has been applied to exempt some activities where the government employee was acting pursuant to a federal statute, regulation, or guideline (Wion, 1989). It is possible that this "discretionary function exception" to FTCA may operate to bar a legal action for research injury against a federal agency such as NIH or FDA. In deciding whether a particular employee's actions qualify under the discretionary function exception, the court will examine whether the employee's actions involved an element of choice or judgment and whether this choice was a permissible exercise of policy judgment (Wion, 1989). If the federal policy is a general one, allowing federal employees some discretion in how

it is implemented, the federal agency may not be sued in tort if the employees' actions result in injury. If the policy is written with detailed requirements, leaving little discretion for federal employees, however, the agency
may be subject to liability if an employee's implementation of that policy
causes injury (Wion, 1989).

The outcome of a legal action for research injury against a federal
agency, such as NIH or FDA, is uncertain. Much of the conduct of research
sponsors and investigators is spelled out in federal policies, but there are
also areas of considerable discretion on the part of federal employees. For
example, in FDA regulations governing new drug applications (NDAs), there
are no product-specific regulations; the regulations contain only general
information about the criteria for approval. Consequently, legal actions against
FDA in connection with NDAs have been dismissed by federal courts under
the discretionary function exception (Wion, 1989). But in one case where
an injured plaintiff claimed FDA made a decision to release a polio vaccine
based on inadequate animal test data, the court held that FDA's assessment
of the animal data was a scientific determination, not the exercise of a
discretionary function, and thus subject to liability (*Griffin v. United States*).
It is not clear whether the particular actions of a researcher/investigator in
implementing federal policy regarding research on human subjects would
be considered a scientific determination or a discretionary policy judgment.

*IRBs and research institutions*    The research institution and its IRB may
also be held liable for approving a negligent protocol or for not closely
monitoring or supervising the ongoing research. Under the tort doctrine of
"respondeat superior," hospitals may be held liable for the negligent activities of their employees (Campbell, 1969). In *Friter v. IOLAB Corporation*,
a Pennsylvania court recently found that a hospital, as a participant in a
clinical investigation for the FDA, had assumed a duty under federal regulations to ensure that informed consent was obtained from research participants.

There have been no reported cases in which IRB members were successfully sued for breaching their duty to protect research subjects, male or
female (Flannery and Greenberg, 1994). Nevertheless, the potential exists
for liability of both IRBs and their individual members. An IRB could be
found negligent, for example, if it approves an informed consent process
later found to be inadequate. Federal policies on informed consent are detailed but leave some discretion to the IRB—for example, whether the research warrants inclusion of a statement about possible unforeseeable risks
to an embryo or fetus. In addition, the regulations permit an IRB to waive
certain elements of the consent form if it determines that only minimal risk
is involved (Bordas, 1984).

Federal regulations require that an IRB ensure that investigators obtain the consent of the participants, but most IRBs trust the investigator to obtain proper consent. Regulations authorize IRB members to observe the consent process, but a 1982 poll found that only 2 out of 100 IRB members had ever required anyone other than the investigator to be involved in the informed consent process (Robertson, 1982).

Given the potential conflict of interest that an investigator brings to the consent process (it is in an investigator's best interest to acquire participants), a court could find that an IRB negligently relied on the investigator if it finds the participant never gave informed consent or was coerced into consenting.

Courts may also find IRBs negligent if they fail to conduct a continuing review of approved research, as required by statute. A 1978 study by the National Commission for the Protection of Human Subjects of Biomedical and Behavioral Research revealed that only half of the IRBs had a policy requiring investigators to report participant injuries; just over a third designated someone to observe a research project; and only half of this group routinely did so (Bordas, 1984). The courts might find that the negligent actions of the investigator were an intervening cause of the injury, absolving the IRB from liability, but if the IRB should have anticipated the actions of the investigator, it can still be found negligent for exposing participants to the risk (Bordas, 1984, citing Prosser, 1971).

If the IRB is part of a state-owned institution, it may be considered an agent of the state. The doctrine of sovereign immunity might bar legal actions against the state, thus protecting the IRB and its members from liability. Some states retain their own sovereign immunity, but over the past few decades the doctrine has been weakened by exceptions. There is also the possibility that members of hospital-based IRBs might be protected by state statutes that provide immunity to members of hospital review committees (Bordas, 1984). Thus, while there is potential for IRBs to be the targets of legal action, both as individuals and as an entity, no IRB has been successfully sued for a research injury, and they may be granted immunity under various state-created immunity doctrines.

### Liability for Injuries to Offspring

As mentioned above, the greatest source of concern about liability is the possibility of injury to offspring when women of childbearing potential are included in clinical drug trials. Fear of liability to offspring may be based on a number of factors. First, the fear is inspired by the experiences of diethylstilbestrol (DES) and thalidomide cases, where offspring were seriously injured by the mother's ingestion of the drug during pregnancy (see Appendix C for DES Case Study). As a result, there is a high level of concern about the inclusion of women of childbearing potential in drug trials, particularly in early phase studies when effects on both adult and offspring are largely unknown. Second, although it may be difficult for a plaintiff to prove causation, the magnitude of harm that could be alleged to result from in utero exposure to a drug is great. Third, the statute of limitations usually is longer for cases of injury to children, and damage that occurs in utero may not show up until years later, leaving potential defendants liable for an indeterminate amount of time. Finally, securing a parent's consent to the research is unlikely to preclude recovery by a child for injuries in utero, because strong arguments can be made that a parent cannot waive a child's rights to sue. The rationale behind such a policy is to avoid conflicts of interest between parents and children (Clayton, 1994; *Apicella v. Valley Forge Military Academy and Junior College*).

*Tort law and prenatal injuries*   Initially, recovery for prenatal injuries was denied because there was no authority for such an action; an unborn child was considered to be part of its mother, without a separate legal existence. This view persisted until 1946, when a federal court in *Bonbrest v. Kotz* held that a child may recover after birth for injuries suffered as a viable fetus. Many states adopted this rule, with the requirements that the child be born alive and that the injury occur when the fetus was viable (*Shack v. Holland*). The viability rule was subsequently abandoned in most jurisdictions, and prenatal injury claims in general now are seen as compensable, sometimes with large damage awards (Clayton, 1994).

Courts have shown some reluctance to recognize a cause of action for preconception injury. It may be difficult for the plaintiff to establish the necessary causal link between the defendant's behavior and the child's injuries. Courts are also uneasy with the notion of extending liability back to before the point of conception, because this greatly expands the boundaries of foreseeable injuries for which a defendant can be held responsible (Merton, 1992). Some states have allowed recovery for preconception injuries, while others have denied recovery.[8] The best-known cases for preconception injury are those of "DES granddaughters," women whose mothers were exposed to DES in utero; nearly all of these claims have been rejected by the courts (Sherman, 1990; *Enright v. Eli Lilly & Co.*). (See Appendix C for more information on the DES cases.)

Potential plaintiffs in a legal action for injuries to offspring include the child, as long as he or she is born alive, and the parents. The tort principle will vary depending on whether the child was born alive and what the parents would have done if they had been adequately informed about risks to offspring. When the plaintiff is the child, the likelihood of a successful legal action depends in part on the ability of the parents to show they would not have participated in the research had they known about the risks. Damage awards to these children can include pain and suffering and damages to cover their special needs over the course of a lifetime (Clayton, 1994; Keeton et al., 1984). If the parents claim, however, that they would not have had the child if they had been informed of the risks, the child's action is one of *wrongful life.* Very few states have recognized such an action (Clayton, 1994).

Parents of a liveborn child who allege that they would not have participated in the research if they had known about the risks may recover the additional medical expenses that are not covered in the damage award from the child's legal action. Most of the time they may not recover for their own pain and suffering, because they are considered to be "bystanders" to their child's injury. If the parents claim that they would not have had a child had they been fully informed of the risks of the research, their action is one for *wrongful birth.* If the child is stillborn as a result of a research injury, the parents may bring an action for *wrongful death;* in states that permit such a cause of action, the damage award is usually relatively small (Clayton, 1994).

*Potential defendants*    In addition to all of the defendants discussed above, it may be possible for the child to sue a parent for participating in a clinical drug trial, depending on the law of parent-child immunity in the state. Under parent-child immunity, children are not permitted to sue their parents. Some states have begun to limit parent-child immunity; others have eliminated it; still others have declared that only some parental decisions will give rise to liability; and a few states retain complete immunity (Clayton, 1994).

Existing case law in this area focuses on the potential of a woman's behavior to result in a bad pregnancy outcome. At least three states have addressed children's claims that they were injured by their mothers' behavior during pregnancy, although none were in the context of research. Two states, Michigan and New Hampshire, permitted the child to recover damages; in one of these cases, the child alleged injury resulting from the mother's ingestion of tetracycline while she was pregnant (*Grodin v. Grodin*; *Bonte v. Bonte*). A third state, Illinois, denied the cause of action, stating that to allow such a claim would intrude too deeply into the lives of pregnant women (*Stallman v. Youngquist*).

For states that allow such recovery, the child must show that the woman was negligent in her behavior—that her choice was one that other reasonable people would not have made. In the research context, this would require an inquiry into whether it was reasonable for the woman to choose to participate in the protocol. According to one commentator, other factors that should be considered include the general deference given to patients to choose their own treatment, the seriousness of the woman's medical problem, and the availability of nonfetotoxic alternatives. The commentator also notes that wrongful life actions—"I should have never been born"—are extremely unlikely to succeed against parents (Clayton, 1994).

In cases where alleged injury to offspring stems from the mother's participation in a drug trial, pharmaceutical manufacturers and the clinical investigators may also be sued. One commentator has suggested that, when the informed consent of the woman was obtained, the third-party defendant may join the woman as a defendant in the action, claiming that she was an intervening cause of the injury or that her choice to participate in the trial was contributory negligence (Merton, 1992). In tort law generally, the presence of an intervening cause may operate to extinguish liability for the other party, but public policy may dictate that a parent not be recognized as an intervening cause in this situation. Another commentator has argued that allowing third-party defendants to escape liability by bringing the woman into the action would contradict the rationale for not allowing parents to release the legal claims of their children (Clayton, 1994). Finally, the court also may seek to have the defendant with greater financial resources be responsible for paying the damages; in most cases this will be a third party rather than a parent.

*Sufficiency of informed consent*   Under the limited case precedent available, the likelihood of a successful legal action for offspring injury has depended on whether obtaining informed consent from the woman is sufficient, in all circumstances, to avoid liability. The committee is aware of emerging data concerning the possibility of male-mediated developmental effects (see Chapter 7); nevertheless, this possibility has not operated to exclude fertile men as a class from clinical drug trials. Hence the committee frames the issue in terms of the woman's participation in clinical trials.

Of all of the reported cases of research injury, only two concerned injuries to offspring. Both cases came out of the University of Chicago experiments with DES in pregnant women, where there was a failure to secure the woman's consent to participate in the research (see Appendix C). There is no case precedent to set the boundaries for liability for injuries to offspring when the woman's valid consent to the research has been secured.

At least one court has held that the informed consent of the woman is sufficient to avoid liability for injury to offspring if the research is a therapeutic intervention for the fetus (*Roberts v. Patel*). The rationale of this one case seems to imply that if the woman has a serious illness and is participating in a clinical trial of a treatment that could be beneficial to her, there will likely be no recovery in tort for injuries to her or to her offspring, as long as there was no negligence involved and the informed consent of the woman was properly secured. The risk of liability may be higher, however, for both the woman and the pharmaceutical company, if the intervention is a benefit to the mother but is not for a serious illness, or if there are safer alternative interventions available *and* the risk to the fetus is known or suspected to be significant.

For trials of drugs that are completely nontherapeutic to either the woman or fetus (for example, early phase trials of drugs where testing is done in healthy participants), the outcome of an offspring injury case is even more unclear. DHHS regulations on research in children may be instructive here. Under the current regulations, in some cases parents may consent for their minor children to be research subjects in protocols that do not directly benefit the children. DHHS may fund such research only where the IRB finds that:

- The risk represents a minor risk over minimal risk.
- The intervention or procedure presents experiences to subjects that are reasonably commensurate with those inherent in their actual or expected medical, dental, psychological, social, or educational situations.
- The intervention or procedure is likely to yield generalizable knowledge about the subjects' disorder or condition that is of vital importance for the understanding or amelioration of the subjects' disorder or condition.
- Adequate provisions are made for soliciting assent of the children and permission of their parents or guardians (45 C.F.R. 46.406). Permission of both parents is required unless one parent is deceased, unknown, incompetent, or not reasonably available, or when only one parent has legal custody of the child (45 C.F.R. 46.408(b)).

For research involving greater than minimal risk, there is no category for research of no benefit to the child; however, the regulations do specify that, for research that would not otherwise be approved but "would present an opportunity to understand, prevent, or alleviate a serious problem affecting the health or welfare of children," the IRB must submit such research to DHHS for approval (45 C.F.R. 46.407). A court may find, however, that these regulations governing research on minors do not apply to offspring injury resulting from a woman's participation in a clinical study.

If a woman consents to participate in a trial where the treatment is not for a serious illness and presents a known or possible significant risk of harm to the fetus, what would be the result? Because there is no legal precedent for such a scenario, the committee can only speculate about the outcome. If the research has been pursued negligently, or the informed consent process was not legally sound, it is possible that the offspring would recover under the same legal principles applicable to medical malpractice, as discussed above.

If there is no negligence, and informed consent of the woman has been properly secured, it may still be possible for the offspring to recover. Because it is the IRB's responsibility to ascertain whether the benefits of a particular research protocol outweigh the risks for any class of potential participants, the IRB could be liable for approving a protocol that permits participation of pregnant women where there is *no* benefit to the woman and some risk to the fetus. At least one commentator has noted that there may be settings where third parties are not entitled to rely on even fully informed consent of the woman to guard against liability, particularly if the protocol poses serious risks to the fetus while offering little benefit to the woman (Clayton, 1994).

Yet another commentator noted that there is no precedent for imposing liability on a researcher who has properly obtained informed consent for harm to a participant's offspring. Because the harm is done by the woman's choice to participate in a research protocol, with full knowledge that it might have damaging consequences, the woman's negligent choice is an intervening cause in the injury (Merton, 1992). There is considerable disagreement over whether a court would find a mother legally liable for injury to offspring resulting from her participation in a clinical trial, but some agreement about the remote likelihood of successful legal action by an injured offspring against a pharmaceutical manufacturer who has obtained valid informed consent from the mother (Reisman, 1992; R. Blumberg, FDA Office of the General Counsel, personal communication, August 1993; Flannery and Greenberg, 1994).

*Consent of the father*[9]    As mentioned above, there may also be risks to offspring when fertile men participate in trials of drugs that may cause damage to germ cells. The issue here, however, is whether the father's consent is necessary to avoid liability for injury to the offspring when the mother participates in a clinical trial of little or no benefit to her and with risk of harm to the fetus. There is no explicit policy or case law, but analogies from related areas may apply. For medical treatment of minors, one parent's informed consent is sufficient (Holder, 1985); DHHS regulations for research on children also require the consent of only one parent. Because the concern is with harm to a fetus rather than a child, federal regulations with respect to fetal tissue research may also be relevant; where such research is permitted, it requires informed consent of both father and mother, unless the father's identity and location cannot reasonably be ascertained, the father is not reasonably available, or the pregnancy resulted from rape (45 C.F.R. § 46.209-210). This committee is concerned with the participation of women in clinical research, however, and thus the case law on abortion, where a woman chooses for her own benefit to undergo a medical procedure, may be more applicable. An earlier section of this chapter discusses how the Supreme Court has invalidated state laws requiring a woman to obtain spousal consent or give spousal notification before obtaining an abortion. Based on these examples, it is unlikely the father's consent could be required in order for a pregnant woman to participate in a clinical trial, or that the addition of the father's consent would shield a manufacturer from liability.

## Is *Johnson Controls* Relevant?

Some commentators have suggested that the language of the recent decision by the Supreme Court in *Johnson Controls*, discussed in the foregoing section on constitutional issues, might be influential in future case decisions in other contexts. While certainly not decisive, it may be pertinent in decisions relating to liability for injuries to offspring from clinical research. The company argued that fear of tort liability justified its policy of excluding women from jobs with potentially high lead exposure. The Court rejected this argument noting that "if, under general tort principles, Title VII bans sex-specific fetal protection policies, the employer fully informs the woman of the risk, and the employer has not acted negligently, the basis for holding an employer liable seems remote at best." Since *Johnson Controls* was a case of employment discrimination, this comment on the unlikelihood of liability is not to be interpreted as definitive, but it may provide support for persons who assert that adequate informed consent from the woman would be sufficient protection against liability.

## Liability for Exclusion

Liability for excluding women from clinical trials may be a serious risk, particularly for pharmaceutical manufacturers and, indirectly, for physicians. Manufacturers' liability results when, after a drug is on the market, evidence emerges that the drug is more dangerous or less effective in women (Flannery and Greenberg, 1994). For example, a woman may have an adverse reaction from one of her prescriptions and discover that the drug was never tested in women. Her injury is not a *research injury* as this term has been used thus far. In this example it is the woman's exclusion from clinical research, not her inclusion, that caused the injury. Increased awareness on the part of women that they are not always represented in the populations tested may contribute to an increasing number of legal actions for exclusion.

Under strict liability principles, manufacturers may be held liable for the defective design of a product, and a drug that has not been adequately tested may be found to be defectively designed (Flannery and Greenberg, 1994). In addition, manufacturers must warn about not only the known risks, but also foreseeable risks that should have been known if "reasonable, developed human skill and foresight" had been applied (Flannery and Greenberg, 1994, quoting ALI, 1977).

The duty to warn about foreseeable risks requires that pharmaceutical manufacturers apply state-of-the-art testing methods to their products. With all of the recent publicity about physiological differences between men and women with regard to drug efficacy, dosing, and adverse reactions, it would be difficult to argue that all-male studies of drugs that may be used by women represent state-of-the-art testing methods (Flannery and Greenberg, 1994). In states with a case-by-case determination of the application of comment k (which protects pharmaceutical manufacturers against strict liability—see above), manufacturers will have a difficult time arguing that a drug is "unavoidably" unsafe if they fail to test the drug in a population that might foreseeably use it (Bowles, 1992). Also, if the courts find that the manufacturer deliberately avoided learning about whether a risk was associated with its drug, the manufacturer could be liable for punitive damages as well (Flannery and Greenberg, 1994).

In contrast to the lack of reported legal cases of injury from inclusion in research, there are a number of cases in which damages were awarded to plaintiffs, in part because of inadequate testing of the drug before it was released into the market. Courts have no qualms about scrutinizing the research design of a clinical trial and criticizing research sponsors, not only for unreliable technique and sloppy data handling but also for a lack of response to actual market conditions (Merton, 1992, citing *Tinnerholm v. Parke, Davis & Co*). In one such case, *West v. Johnson & Johnson Products, Inc.*, a woman who claimed that she had suffered from toxic shock syndrome resulting from use of a tampon marketed by Johnson & Johnson Products was awarded damages. The court found that the company had failed to study the basic microbiology of the human vagina, to test for vaginal infections, and to include women with a history of vaginitis in their human studies (Merton, 1992). In *Taylor v. Wyeth Laboratories*, the court found that a prudent manufacturer, once aware that women with type A blood experience a disproportionate number of pulmonary embolisms, would have looked at the relationship between blood type and blood-clotting risk in women taking oral contraceptives (Merton, 1992). Courts have also awarded damages to injured plaintiffs on the grounds of inadequate testing for adverse effects, even in cases where the FDA did not require further testing (Merton, 1992, citing *Barson v. E.R. Squibb & Sons, Inc.*).

In legal actions where the plaintiff claims inadequacy of premarket testing, however, plaintiffs may face some difficulty in proving that their injuries were caused by a failure to test for foreseeable risks. In *Jones v. Ortho Pharmaceutical Corp.*, the plaintiff sought to hold Ortho liable for her carcinoma in situ, claiming that they failed to conduct clinical trials that would have established whether the oral contraceptive she took caused cancer. Because a tort action must prove that the defendant's behavior caused the injury, the plaintiff attempted to persuade the court that because Ortho did not conduct the proper clinical trials, which would have enabled her to show the causal link between the contraceptive and her cancer, the company was presumptively liable. The California intermediate appellate court would not allow the plaintiff to presume causation from a lack of premarket testing (Merton, 1992).

Thus, although there is a general lack of case law on liability for injuries to research participants, there is some precedent for liability for exclusion from research. The case law suggests that if a drug was found to cause injuries to women, and yet women had been excluded from clinical trials of the drug, the pharmaceutical manufacturer might be held liable for failing to test the drug in women. For some drugs, however, the potential for teratogenic or mutagenic effects is low or the negative effects are manifested after a long latent period. For these drugs, even adequate testing in all relevant populations may not reveal their potential to cause harm. At least one commentator has noted that establishing surveillance systems, or requiring companies to keep track of and report adverse drug reactions, may provide plaintiffs with a source of evidence that a company knew or should have known that a particular drug or dose level was potentially dangerous and required further testing or a more adequate warning label (Gibbs and Mackler, 1987).

For physicians, liability resulting from exclusion of women from drug trials arises in the form of negligent drug prescription. For example, the physician could be liable for prescribing a drug to a woman: (1) for a different purpose than that for which it was initially designed and tested or (2) in disregard of the drug's label that it has not been tested in women. With regard to liability for offspring injury resulting from exclusion of women (or men) from drug trials, information about testing for reproductive and developmental effects is often not available for all drugs for which such testing would be appropriate.

## CONCLUSIONS AND RECOMMENDATIONS

The many federal regulations governing research on human subjects do not provide investigators and IRBs with clear answers on issues concerning the inclusion of women and racial and ethnic groups in clinical studies. Recent changes in policies, however, have made them more consistent. All of the recent changes have been implemented to promote the inclusion rather than exclusion of women. Consistency and, where possible, congruence among these policies is important to promote compliance and prevent confusion.

Policies and regulations issued by the FDA or other PHS agencies must be harmonized with those of NIH. At the very least, policies and regulations issued by NIH and those issued by FDA must not be contradictory. The closer the congruence between FDA and NIH regulations and policies, the more likely that a regulated institution will understand precisely what is required and be motivated to comply. When NIH updated its policy concerning inclusion of women in 1991, and added the sanction of possible reduction in the project's priority score for noncompliance, many in the research community came to believe that FDA and NIH policies were contradictory. Now that the FDA has updated its 1977 policy, and NIH is in the process of updating its 1991 policy, there is an opportunity to achieve congruence between the positions of the two agencies.

**The committee recommends that NIH work closely with the FDA and with other PHS agencies to make regulations and policies on inclusion of women and racial and ethnic groups consistent with one another and, wherever possible, to make them congruent.**

If the policies of the two agencies are harmonized, there will still remain the task of educating the research community concerning what is required, and motivating that community to comply. Enunciation of sound and congruent policies, in conjunction with a comprehensive educational program, will ensure that policies and the rationales for the policies are properly understood by the research community.

**The committee recommends that NIH, in cooperation with FDA, should institute a comprehensive education program directed at investigators, institutions and IRBs on policies concerning the inclusion of women and racial and ethnic groups in clinical studies.**

It is impossible to quantify the risk of tort liability from the inclusion of women in clinical studies at this time, because: (1) there is no complete compendium of unreported cases involving settlements and (2) women have not been included in some major studies in the past. Difficulties of prediction are compounded because tort law is governed by the individual states, with many variations on issues such as whether a woman's informed consent will serve to bar an independent action by a child injured as a fetus during such research. Analysis of existing legal rules and principles seems to indicate that the likelihood of successful damage actions is limited. Nevertheless, broadening the research population to include those groups previously excluded may also generate additional legal actions that will test existing legal doctrine.

A special set of concerns in the research area stems from the differing bases for liability according to which party is a defendant. A pharmaceutical company, for example, might be sued on the basis of strict liability, while a researcher ordinarily would be sued only on the basis of negligence.

With regard to the latter, the new federal policies calling for inclusion of women in clinical studies will help establish new standards that will be relevant to legal actions.

Many of the concerns voiced about liability in the context of research including women are the same as those with regard to the tort system in general. For example, expert scientific testimony is necessary to establish that a particular drug caused an injury. There are inherent difficulties in assuring the unbiased nature of such testimony in what are often highly technical cases.

**The committee recommends that current and future initiatives toward general tort reform include attention to issues of research-related injury, including issues of proof of causation.**

The question of whether there should be a special compensation scheme for injuries sustained by children as a result of a parent's participation in a clinical study is similar to that raised in the context of research subjects in general. The committee does not recommend adoption—at this time—of a special compensation scheme limited to coverage of children injured prenatally or preconceptually. Any new compensation scheme focusing only on such injuries poses especially difficult problems with regard to establishing causation and averting large numbers of questionable recoveries. Appendix D discusses several existing compensation schemes dealing with children and illustrates these and other difficulties.

**The committee recommends that NIH thoroughly review the area of compensation for research injury in general and that consideration of implementation of any compensation scheme include attention to prenatal and preconceptual injuries to children resulting from a parent's participation in a clinical study.**

Our current health care reimbursement system does not include coverage for medical care resulting from injuries sustained during research. This could be accomplished through a system of universal access with adequate coverage.

**The committee recommends that health care reform efforts include considerations of medical care for research-related injury.**

The committee recognizes that, regardless of their basis or justification, fears about liability are real. On balance, however, the committee concludes that liability concerns should not represent an impediment to implementation of public policies that favor the broader inclusion of women in clinical studies.

## NOTES

1. Department of Agriculture, Department of Energy, National Aeronautics and Space Administration, Department of Commerce, Consumer Product Safety Commission, International Development Cooperating Agency, Agency for International Development, Department of Housing and Urban Development, Department of Justice, Department of Defense, Department of Education, Department of Veterans Affairs, Environmental Protection Agency, Department of Health and Human Services, National Science Foundation, Department of Transportation.

2. Previously, in *Planned Parenthood of Central Missouri v. Danforth,* the Supreme Court invalidated a state law requiring a woman to obtain consent of her spouse before obtaining an abortion. The Court stated that "Inasmuch as it is the woman who physically bears the child and who is the more directly and immediately affected by the pregnancy, as between the two, the balance weighs in her favor."

3. One notable exception is *In re A.C.,* where the appellate court overturned the decision of the trial court to force a woman to undergo a caesarean in order to save her baby. The court held that "in virtually all cases the question of what is to be done is to be decided by the patient—the pregnant woman—on behalf of herself and the fetus" (*In re A.C.*).

4. See the paper by Professor Debra DeBruin in Volume 2 of this report for further analysis of whether women are owed affirmative action measures as a result of past discrimination in research.

5. In the one case in which NIH was the defendant, which the general counsel's office believes was dismissed, a prisoner claimed he was due credit for good behavior for participating in a study. In the other two, an NIH grantee institution was the defendant. In one, a prisoner claimed participation an NIH-funded study as defense to murder (he received a defective batch of experimental human growth hormone as a child); in the second, the plaintiff, who had a suicidal history, sued for improper care and monitoring after he jumped out of the window while on an experimental epilepsy drug (personal communication, S. Sherman, Associate General Counsel, NIH, June 1993).

6. At least one attorney for a pharmaceutical company has commented that it may not be the reality of the liability but the perception of legal risk that causes many drug companies to take defensive action to avoid possible involvement in a legal proceeding (IOM, 1991b).

7. The Supreme Court recently rejected the long-standing *Frye* rule, which set the standard for the acceptability of scientific evidence in legal proceedings. The *Frye* rule required that any proposed scientific testimony must have received general acceptance of its reliability by the relevant scientific community before the court would admit it into evidence. In *Daubert*

*v. Merrell Dow Pharmaceuticals*, the Court explained that *Frye*'s general acceptance standard was superseded by the adoption of the Federal Rules of Evidence. Under the Federal Rules, the trial judge makes a flexible determination of whether the evidence rests on a reliable foundation and is relevant to the task at hand. The effect this change in evidentiary rules will have on the liability climate for research injuries is unknown.

8. See *Bergstrasser v. Mitchell* (court allowed a child to recover for damages caused by his premature birth, which allegedly resulted from a previous negligently performed C-section); *Renslow v. Mennonite Hospital* (court allowed infant to recover for injury caused by a negligent blood transfusion of the mother before conception); *Monusko v. Postle*; *Albala v. City of New York*.

9. "Father" is the term chosen here to include the biological father of the baby, the child's legal guardian, or anyone the law would recognize as having legal responsibility for the welfare of a child.

## REFERENCES

ALI (American Law Institute). 1977. Restatement (Second) of Torts Section 402A.

Bordas, L.M. 1984. Note: Tort liability of institutional review boards. *West Virginia Law Review* 87:137-164.

Bowles, L.E. 1992. The disenfranchisement of fertile women in clinical trials: The legal ramifications of and solutions for rectifying the knowledge gap. *Vanderbilt Law Review* 45(4):877-920.

Bush, J.K. 1993. Women's participation in clinical research: The industry perspective. Presented at Conference on the Inclusion of Women and Minorities in Clinical Research, Bethesda, Md., June 28, 1993.

Caban, C. 1993. Personal communication with T. Johnson. May 7. (Dr. Carlos Caban advises the NIH Office of Research on Women's Health with respect to its policy on the inclusion of women in clinical research.)

Campbell, J.E. 1969. Civil Liability for Investigational Drugs: Part II. *Temple Law Quarterly* 42(4):289-354.

Cardon, P.V., Dommel, F.W., Jr., and Trumble, R.R. 1976. Injuries to research subjects: A survey of investigators. *New England Journal of Medicine* 295:650-654.

Charo, R.A. 1994. Constitutional issues raised by the exclusion of women from research trials. In: Women and Health Research: Ethical and Legal Issues of Including Women in Clinical Studies, Volume 2, A. Mastroianni, R. Faden, and D. Federman, eds. Washington, D.C.: National Academy Press.

Clayton, E.W. 1994. Liability exposure when offspring are injured because of their parents' participation in clinical trials. In: Women and Health Research: Ethical and Legal Issues of Including Women in Clinical Studies, Volume 2, A. Mastroianni, R. Faden, and D. Federman, eds. Washington, D.C.: National Academy Press.

Department of the Army. 1992. Memorandum from Gregory P. Berezuk, Chief, Human Use Review and Regulatory Affairs Office, Office of the Surgeon General, re: Human subjects research review board policy regarding pregnancy testing of research subjects (January 21).

Department of Energy. 1992. Protecting Human Research Subjects at the Department of

Energy: Human Subjects Handbook. Washington, D.C.: Office of Health and Environ-
     mental Research, Office of Energy Research, Department of Energy.
Department of Veterans Affairs. 1992. Inclusion of women and minorities in clinical research.
     Veterans Health Administration Manual M-3, Part 1, Chapter 14 (July 24).
Flannery, E., and Greenberg, S.N. 1994. Liability exposure for exclusion and inclusion of
     women as subjects in clinical studies. In: Women and Health Research: Ethical and Legal
     Issues of Including Women in Clinical Studies, Volume 2, A. Mastroianni, R. Faden, and
     D. Federman, eds. Washington, D.C.: National Academy Press.
FDA (Food and Drug Administration). 1993. Guideline for the study and evaluation of gender
     differences in the clinical evaluation of drugs. Notice. *Federal Register* 58(139):39406-
     39416.
FDA. 1977. General Consideration for the Clinical Evaluation of Drugs. Rockville, Md.: FDA.
Gibbs, J.N., and Mackler, B.F. 1987. Food and Drug Administration regulation and products
     liability: Strong sword, weak shield. *Tort and Insurance Law Journal* 22(Winter):194-
     243.
Green, V. 1993. Doped Up, Knocked Up, and Locked Up?: The Criminal Prosecution of
     Women Who Use Drugs During Pregnancy. New York: Garland.
Harvard Medical Practice Study. 1990. Patients, doctors, and lawyers: Studies of medical
     injury, malpractice litigation, and patient compensation in New York. Boston: Harvard
     Medical Practice Study.
Holder, A.R. 1985. Legal Issues in Pediatrics and Adolescent Medicine. New Haven: Yale
     University Press.
IOM (Institute of Medicine). 1989. Medical Professional Liability and the Delivery of Obstet-
     rical Care. Washington, D.C.: National Academy Press.
IOM. 1991a. Issues in the Inclusion of Women in Clinical Trials. Report of Planning Panel of
     the Institute of Medicine's Division of Health Sciences Policy. March 1-2. Washington,
     D.C.: Institute of Medicine.
IOM. 1991b. Expanding Access to Investigational Therapies for HIV Infection and AIDS.
     Summary of a Conference, March 12-13, 1990. Washington, D.C.: National Academy
     Press.
IOM. 1993. Inclusion of Women in Clinical Trials: Policies for Population Subgroups. Wash-
     ington, D.C.: National Academy Press.
Keeton, W.P., Dobbs, D.B., Keeton, R.E., and Owen, D.G., eds. 1984. Prosser and Keeton on
     the Law of Torts. St. Paul, Minn.: West.
Kinney, E.L., Trautmann, J., Gold, J., Vesell, E.S., and Zelis, R. 1981. Underrepresentation of
     women in new drug trials. *Annals of Internal Medicine* 95(4):495-499.
Kobasic, D.M. 1988. Institutional review boards in the university setting: Review of pharma-
     ceutical testing protocols, informed consent and ethical concerns. *Journal of College and
     University Law* 15(2):185-216.
Mariner, W.K. 1994. Compensation for research injury. In: Women and Health Research:
     Ethical and Legal Issues of Including Women in Clinical Studies, Volume 2, A. Mastroianni,
     R. Faden, and D. Federman, eds. Washington, D.C.: National Academy Press.
Merton, V. 1992. The Exclusion of Pregnant, Pregnable, and Once-Pregnable People a.k.a.
     women) from Biomedical Research. Unpublished Paper (December 12).
Merton, V. 1994. The impact of current relevant federal regulations on the inclusion of female
     subjects in clinical studies. In: Women and Health Research: Ethical and Legal Issues of
     Including Women in Clinical Studies, Volume 2, A. Mastroianni, R. Faden, and D. Federman,
     eds. Washington, D.C.: National Academy Press.
NIH (National Institutes of Health). 1990. NIH Instruction and Information Memorandum OER
     90-5. December 11.
NIH, Office of Research on Women's Health. 1991. National Institutes of Health: Opportuni-

ties for Research on Women's Health. Summary report of a conference held at Hunt Valley, Md., September 4-6.

NIH. 1992. NIH Data Book 1992: Basic Data Relating to the National Institutes of Health. Bethesda, Md.: NIH.

NIH and ADAMHA (Alcohol, Drug Abuse, and Mental Health Administration). 1990. NIH/ADAMHA Policy Concerning Inclusion of Women in Study Populations. *NIH Guide* 19(31):18-19.

NOW Legal Defense and Education Fund. 1992. Citizens' Petition to the FDA, signed by AIDS Service Center HIV Law Project, NOW Legal Defense and Education Fund, and American Civil Liberties Union, AIDS Project. December 15.

NRC (National Research Council). 1989. Biologic Markers in Reproductive Toxicology. Washington, D.C.: National Academy Press.

NRC (National Research Council)/IOM. 1990. Developing New Contraceptives: Obstacles and Opportunities. L. Mastroianni, Jr., P.J. Donaldson, and T.P. Kane, eds. Washington, D.C.: National Academy Press.

PMA (Pharmaceutical Manufacturers Association). 1992. 1992 survey report: 91 medicines in testing; 3 approved this past year. P. 8 in Development: AIDS Medicines, Drugs and Vaccines. Washington, D.C.: PMA.

Rall, J.E. 1990. Memorandum to scientific directors, clinical directors, chiefs, and ICD clinical branches/laboratories from NIH deputy director for intramural research. Policy on the Inclusion of Women in Study Populations: Intramural and Epidemiological (August 1). Bethesda, Md.: National Institutes of Health.

Reisman, E.K. 1992. Products liability: What is the current situation and will it change (and how) when more women are included in studies? Presented at the Women in Clinical Trials of FDA-Regulated Products Workshop, Food and Drug Law Institute, Washington, D.C., October 5.

Robertson, J.A. 1982. The law of institutional review boards. *UCLA Law Review* 25:484-549.

Robertson, J. 1994. Ethical issues related to the inclusion of pregnant women in clinical trials (I). Women and Health Research: Ethical and Legal Issues of Including Women in Clinical Studies, Volume 2, A. Mastroianni, R. Faden, and D. Federman, eds. Washington, D.C.: National Academy Press.

Selwitz, A.S., and Wermeling, D.P. 1992. IRB Policies and Practices: Review of Subject Population. Paper commissioned by the Office of Protection from Research Risks, National Institutes of Health.

Sherman, R. 1990. New DES front. *The National Law Journal* 12(March 12):1, 26-27.

Steinbock, B. 1994. Ethical issues related to the inclusion of pregnant women in clinical trials (II). Women and Health Research: Ethical and Legal Issues of Including Women in Clinical Studies, Volume 2, A. Mastroianni, R. Faden, and D. Federman, eds. Washington, D.C.: National Academy Press.

Tribe, L.H. 1987. American Constitutional Law. Westbury, N.Y.: Foundation Press.

Tribe, L.H. 1991. Abortion: The Clash of Absolutes. New York: W.W. Norton.

U.S. Congress. 1993. House Report 103-28:84.

Wadlington, W. 1984. Breaking the silence of doctor and patient (review of J. Katz's The Silent World of Doctor and Patient). *The Yale Law Journal* 93(8):1640-1651.

Wion, A.H. 1989. Potential implications of the Supreme Court's decision in *Berkovitz v. United States. Food, Drug & Cosmetic Law Journal* 44:145-156.

Wittes, B., and Wittes, J. 1993. Group therapy. *The New Republic* April 5:15-17.

## STATUTES AND REGULATIONS

45 C.F.R. 46
21 C.F.R. 50 & 56
28 U.S.C. § 1346(b), 2674 (19764)
Federal Employees Liability Reform and Tort Compensation Act of 1988, P.L. 15-11

## CASE REFERENCES

*Albala v. City of New York*, 445 N.Y.S. 2d 108 (1981)

*Apicella v. Valley Forge Military Academy and Junior College*, 630 F. Supp. 20 (E.D. Pa. 1985)

*Barson v. E.R. Squibb & Sons, Inc.*, 682 P.2d 832 (Utah 1984)

*Bergstrasser v. Mitchell*, 448 F. Supp. 10 (D.C. Mo. 1977), *aff'd*, 577 F.2d 22 (8th Cir. 1978)

*Bonbrest v. Kotz*, 65 F. Supp. 138 (1946)

*Bonte v. Bonte*, 616 A.2d 464 (N.H. 1992)

*Craig v. Boren*, 429 U.S. 190 (1976)

*Cruzan v. Director, Missouri Department of Health*, 497 U.S. 261 (1990)

*Daubert v. Merrell Dow Pharmaceuticals*, 113 S.Ct. 2786 (1993)

*Enright v. Eli Lilly & Co.*, 570 N.E.2d 198 (N.Y. 1988)

*Friter v. IOLAB Corporation*, 607 A.2d 1111 (Pa. Super. Ct. 1992)

*Gaston v. Hunter*, 588 P.2d 326 (Ariz. Ct. App. 1978)

*Geduldig v. Aiello*, 417 U.S. 484 (1974)

*Griffin v. United States*, 500 F.2d 1949 (3d Cir. 1974)

*Grodin v. Grodin*, 301 N.W.2d 869 (Mich. Ct. App. 1981)

*In re A.C.*, 573 A.2d 1235 (D.C. Ct. App. 1990)

*International Union, UAW v. Johnson Controls*, 111 S. Ct. 1196 (1991)

*Jones v. Ortho Pharmaceutical Corp.*, 209 Cal. Rptr. 456 (1985)

*Monusko v. Postle*, 175 Mich. App. 269, 437 N.W. 2d 367 (1989)

*Newport News Shipping & Dry Dock Co. v. EEOC*, 462 U.S. 669 (1983)

*Personnel Administrator of Massachusetts v. Feeney*, 442 U.S. 256 (1979)

*Planned Parenthood of Central Missouri v. Danforth*, 428 U.S. 52 (1976)

*Planned Parenthood of Southeastern Pennsylvania v. Casey*, 112 S.Ct. 2791 (1992)

*Renslow v. Mennonite Hospital*, 67 Ill.2d 348, 367 N.E. 2d 1250 (1977)

*Roberts v. Patel*, 620 F. Supp. 323 (N.D. Ill. 1985)

*Roe v. Wade*, 410 U.S. 113 (1973)

*Salgo v. Leland Stanford Jr. University*, 317 P.2d 170 (Cal. Ct. App. 1957)

*Shack v. Holland*, 389 N.Y.S.2d 988 (1976)

*Stallman v. Youngquist*, 531 N.E.2d 355 (Ill. 1988)

*Taylor v. Wyeth Laboratories*, 362 N.W.2d 293 (Mich. App. 1984)

*Tinnerholm v. Parke, Davis & Co.*, 285 F. Supp. 432 (S.D.N.Y. 1968), *modified on other grounds*, 411 F.2d 48 (2d Cir. 1969)

*United States v. Orleans*, 425 U.S. 807 (1976)

*West v. Johnson & Johnson Products, Inc.*, 220 Cal.Rptr. 437 (1985)

*Whitlock v. Duke University* 637 F. Supp. 1463 (M.D.N.C. 1986), *aff'd*, 829 F.2d 1340 (4th Cir. 1987)

# 7

# Risks to Reproduction and Offspring

The preceding chapters have identified scientific, social, ethical, and legal issues that would need to be taken into account in implementing the committee's three fundamental principles of justice with regard to the inclusion of women in clinical studies (see Chapter 3). This chapter illustrates these issues, and potential mechanisms for resolving them, with regard to a particular subpopulation—subjects of reproductive age—in a particular category of clinical studies—clinical trials of drugs. Historically, concern for these risks has focused on women of reproductive potential, including pregnant and lactating women. Nevertheless, the possibility that certain drugs pose unique risks to the male reproductive system may also merit attention.

People of reproductive age get sick and take medications, and drugs intended for use by this population should therefore be tested in this population. Some of these drugs, however, have potential risks to reproduction or for the development of offspring. These risks give added importance to informed consent and contraceptive options. Risk assessment for reproductive and developmental toxicity is complicated by the high background rates of infertility and birth defects, as well as the difficulty of identifying the specific effects of the drug under investigation. Techniques such as animal studies, in vitro analysis, and surveillance for developmental effects, among others, can provide some information on potential hazards to humans.

Once the potential reproductive and developmental hazards of participation in a clinical study have been identified, investigators can attempt to design trials to minimize these hazards. In some cases, hazards may be altogether avoidable; in others, it may be decided that hazards cannot be effectively minimized and that the trial should not proceed. The process of weighing potential risks against potential benefits is a complicated process with many players, including the investigator who proposes a study, the institutional review board (IRB) that assures that the protocol is consistent with human subjects regulations, and the potential study participants. This chapter describes some of the factors—such as toxicity data, subjects' understanding of risks, and contraception—that investigators must consider when they wish to study a drug in populations of reproductive age. It also describes the process of making risk-benefit assessments and the values that different people place on certain risks and benefits. The chapter concludes with the committee's recommendations for the conduct of research, including drug trials in persons of reproductive age and in lactating and pregnant women, and a discussion of the policy implications of these recommendations.

## SCIENTIFIC ISSUES: RISK ASSESSMENT

For men and women of reproductive age, and for pregnant and lactating women, there are risks associated with taking experimental and nonexperimental drugs. In many cases, these risks are virtually impossible to detect before the drug is in widespread use because of the inherent limitations of animal studies and clinical trials. Nevertheless, concerns about reproductive and developmental toxicity do not override the need to improve the medical management of these populations. Our understanding of treatment options for all of these groups will only be advanced by their inclusion in clinical studies and by more systematic collection of empirical data on reproductive and developmental outcomes.

### Identifying Reproductive and Developmental Toxicants

Reproductive and developmental toxicants are physical, chemical, and biological agents that produce a toxic effect in animals and/or humans. *Reproductive* toxicants alter fecundity, decreasing the ability or increasing the time needed to achieve pregnancy. *Developmental* toxicants alter the structure or function of offspring. Animal testing and clinical trials are the principal mechanisms for identifying drugs as either reproductive or developmental toxicants. The goal of these approaches is to determine the potential for reproductive and developmental toxicity prior to broader human exposure. In the absence of data from such experimentation, reports of adverse events in humans are also gathered in registries in an attempt to identify unrecognized toxicity. In addition, newborn infants are frequently screened for birth defects so that drugs and other agents with developmental toxicity might be identified.

To determine whether or not a drug is a *potential* human reproductive or developmental toxicant requires two steps: (1) hazard identification and (2) hazard characterization. Characterization of the *magnitude* of the risk for adverse outcome requires two additional steps: (3) exposure assessment and (4) qualitative or quantitative risk characterization (NRC, 1983). Together, these four steps provide the framework for the assessment of risk to reproduction or offspring during a clinical trial.

## Hazard Identification

The first step in risk assessment explores the question: Does the drug produce adverse effects on reproduction or offspring in animals or humans? Because data on the effects of drugs on human reproduction or pregnancy outcome are generally not available prior to a clinical trial, it is necessary to utilize data from animal studies or other studies, such as in vitro assays. Reproductive studies in animals are generally useful and valid for determining whether a drug represents a potential human reproductive or developmental toxicant (Wilson and Fraser, 1979; Shepard, 1983; Schardein, 1985; Jelovsek et al., 1989; Jelovsek et al., 1990). Laboratory animals and humans can differ in toxicokinetics, however, and the use of data from animals to determine health risks in humans must be assessed carefully (NRC, 1989).

## Hazard Characterization

If a drug represents a potential hazard for reproduction or development, it is necessary to determine the dose-response relationship, site of action, and mechanisms through which the adverse effects are produced. Some drugs that appear to be reproductive or developmental toxicants in animals may not produce adverse effects in humans during a clinical trial. For example, compounds metabolized to toxicants in animals may produce different metabolites in humans, or substantially smaller amounts of the same metabolites, and therefore may not represent a hazard. The converse situation also occurs: a chemical may be non-toxic in the conventional animal assays, but be a human developmental toxicant. Fortunately, this is unusual—all known human teratogens are also teratogens in at least one animal species (Schardein, 1985). In addition, genetic differences among humans in their response to toxicants, such as that observed with hydantoin developmental toxicity (Phelan et al., 1982), may also modify risk to reproduction and development.

## Exposure Definition

A critical step in characterizing risk is to define the exposure, including such variables as dose, duration, and timing of exposure with respect to reproduction or pregnancy. For example, exposures that occur before or after the development of a susceptible tissue or organ may carry no additional risk for fetal development. In the case of diethylstilbestrol (DES), the risk of vaginal adenosis is greater than 70 percent for female offspring exposed before the ninth week of gestation but less than 10 percent for exposure after the seventeenth week (see Appendix C). Similarly, in the sexually mature male, exposures to developmental toxicants that occur long before the development of the particular sperm cell that will fertilize an egg are unlikely to affect the development of the resulting offspring, due to the fact that sperm development occurs only in the few months prior to ejaculation.

## Risk Characterization

Finally, after a reproductive or developmental hazard has been identified and characterized, and exposure has been defined, this information is analyzed using statistical models to characterize the risk to reproduction or pregnancy outcome. In this step it is important to define the amount and quality of the data available to characterize risk, including variability and uncertainty in the risk estimate. The risk characterization should also include the assessment of the background incidence of adverse reproductive or developmental outcomes.

## Challenges to Identification of Reproductive and Developmental Toxicants

In order to isolate and evaluate observed drug effects, it is also necessary to consider the background incidence of adverse reproductive or developmental outcomes. This incidence is often higher than many potential study subjects would suppose. For example, about 15 percent of couples trying to conceive will not have done so after one year of trying (a common definition of infertility); 20 to 30 percent of recognized pregnancies end in miscarriage; 3 to 8 percent of all babies have birth defects; and 1 percent of liveborn children are born with severe mental retardation. Most of these adverse outcomes do not have recognized causes, and very few of those with known causes are the result of exposures to chemical, physical, or biologic agents.

With such a high background rate of many different adverse outcomes, identification of adverse effects imposed by a specific drug exposure can be difficult. For example, consider an exposure that increases the incidence of limb reduction defects tenfold. If the baseline incidence of such defects is 1 in 10,000 (0.01 percent), the impact of an increase to 0.1 percent will be undetectable against a background incidence of total birth defects of about 5 percent. It is only when there is some idea of the kind of defect associated with the exposure that studies can be targeted at detecting an increase in incidence.

Determining whether a drug or other treatment is associated with an adverse reproductive or developmental effect also requires characterization of the endpoint of concern. Depending on the endpoint in question, sample sizes required to detect that endpoint can vary greatly (see Table 7-1). An uncommon endpoint such as a rare congenital malformation typically requires very large study populations: a malformation that occurs in only 1 of 10,000 births may not be detected in a trial involving 5,000 couples. When exposure produces a dramatic increase in the incidence of unusual abnormalities, however, it may not take very many cases before the association is recognized. This kind of recognition occurred, for example, with the birth defects associated with thalidomide and isotretinoin, with the cerebral-palsy-like illness caused by methyl mercury, and with the severe testicular toxicity of the pesticide dibromochloropropane (DBCP).

Determining whether or not a drug is associated with a relatively common adverse outcome such as miscarriage may be defined with a much smaller number of subjects. Listed in Table 7-1 are some adverse reproductive and developmental outcomes of interest, the background rate of these adverse outcomes, and the sample size needed to determine a doubling of that outcome in a clinical trial.

## Male-Mediated Developmental Toxicity

Although traditional concerns about developmental toxicity have focused on exposures (or treatment) of the female during pregnancy, scientists have long suspected that the male may also contribute to adverse pregnancy outcomes such as spontaneous abortion, stillbirth, impaired growth, and structural and functional abnormalities (Olshein and Mattison, in press). Most systematic studies of male-mediated developmental toxicity, however, have been rodent studies, and the implications are inconclusive for human males.

Scientists have postulated that the occurrence of developmental toxicity following exposure or treatment of the male may depend on a number of factors, including male reproductive status (fecundity), exposure (dose, duration), properties of the agent, pharmacokinetics (especially distribution to gonads and other endocrine organs), mechanism of action, stage of spermatogenesis affected, frequency and timing of intercourse with respect to

TABLE 7-1  Expected Frequency of Selected Endpoints of Reproductive or Developmental Failure and the Sample Size Needed to Detect a Doubling of that Endpoint in a Clinical Trial

| Reproductive or Developmental Endpoint | Denominator | Frequency (%)[a] | Sample Size of Treatment and Control Groups to Detect a Doubling of the Endpoint[b] |
|---|---|---|---|
| Azospermia | Men | 1 | 3,300 Men |
| Failure to conceive after one year of unprotected intercourse | Couples | 10-15 (12) | 230 Couples |
| Birth weight <2,500 g | Live births | 5-15 (10) | 286 Live births |
| Miscarriage | Pregnancies | 10-20 (15) | 174 Pregnancies |
| Chromosome aberration at miscarriage | Miscarriages | 40-50 (45) | 25 Miscarriages |
| Late fetal deaths (≥28 weeks) | Late fetal deaths + live births | 1-4 (3) | 1,068 Late fetal deaths + live births |
| Total birth defects at birth | Live births | 2-3 (3) | 1,068 Live births |
| Chromosome aberrations at birth | Live births | 0.6 | 5,533 Live births |
| Neural tube defects | Late fetal deaths + live births | 0.005-1 (0.05) | 66,936 Late fetal deaths + live births |
| Severe mental retardation | Children to age 15 | 0.4 | 8,324 Children to age 15 |

[a]Where a range is given, the background rate used in the determination of sample size is shown in parentheses.

[b]The sample size indicated is the size required of each population (i.e., both the study population and the control population will need to be at least as large as the sample size indicated) to detect a doubling in the rate of the indicated endpoint. In these calculations it is assumed that the control and study populations are the same size, and that the investigator wants a 90 percent chance to detect a statistically significant difference in the study and control populations at a $p \leq 0.05$. The calculations were performed with the sample size estimation modules for an unmatched comparison of proportions as implemented in True Epistat 4.0, Epistat Services, Richardson, Texas (1991). The function for the sample size calculation for unpaired comparison of proportions is described on page 399 of Zar, 1984.

TABLE 7-2  Adverse Developmental Effects that May Occur Following
Male Exposure

| Reproductive Process | Toxicological Effect of Male Exposure | Endpoint Observed in Epidemiological Studies |
| --- | --- | --- |
| Conception | Preimplantation loss | Decreased fertility<br>Increased time to pregnancy |
| Implantation | Postimplantation loss | Increased spontaneous abortion |
| Embryo development | Failure/disruption of embryonic development | Increased spontaneous abortion<br>Increased fetal death<br>Increased malformation<br>Increased growth retardation<br>Increased functional deficit<br>Increased premature birth |
| Fetal growth and development | Failure/disruption of fetal growth and development | Increased fetal death<br>Increased malformation<br>Increased growth retardation<br>Increased premature birth<br>Increased functional deficit |

exposure, and maternal reproductive characteristics (fecundity). In addition, the type of endpoint that is observed is likely to vary with the process affected in the male (see Table 7-2). Studies conducted over the past five decades have identified three potential mechanisms of male-mediated developmental toxicity:

1. *Genetic:* damage to the genetic material contained in the sperm through the creation of a mutation or chromosomal abnormality.
2. *Epigenetic:* damage to processes that control the expression of the paternal genes after fertilization.
3. *Transport of toxicant:* transport of an agent through the ejaculate during postconception sexual intercourse and subsequent exposure of the conceptus, embryo, or fetus.

Although evidence is inconclusive concerning the role of the male in developmental toxicity, the possibility that he has a role provides reason enough for investigators to consider including discussion of developmental toxicity in the informed consent process for male subjects who may be exposed to developmental toxicants in the course of a clinical study. As discussed below, the provision of advice about contraceptive options may also be wise.

### Evaluating Drugs for Use in Men and Women of Reproductive Age

Women of reproductive age (defined as 15 to 44 years of age) constitute a significant proportion of the population. Men of reproductive age constitute an even greater proportion, because the window of potential fertility is much larger for males. Not surprisingly, members of this large segment of the population experience a myriad of diseases requiring medical treatment, and drugs intended for use in this population should be tested in this population. As discussed in earlier chapters, federal policies and practices designed to protect women of reproductive potential from risks associated with experimental treatment have hindered the collection of information about drug effects in this subpopulation.

Investigators designing clinical studies need to be particularly concerned about the potential reproductive and developmental toxicity of the compounds they wish to study in this population. When a trial involves the exposure to a potential toxicant, issues of risk characterization, informed consent, and contraceptive options are paramount. Because people tend to overestimate the risks of harm to reproduction and development that are posed by drugs (Koren et al., 1989, 1990), enhanced subject education efforts may be required. Other characteristics of the population of reproductive age, such as use of hormonal contraceptives, must also be taken into account during trial design and recruitment. Discussed in greater detail below are the kinds of variables that investigators must consider when deciding how best to test new drugs in men and women of reproductive age.

### Use of Toxicity Testing Data

If information is available on the reproductive and developmental effects of a given drug in animals, investigators must make several types of inferences in order to protect the reproductive and developmental health of their subjects (see Figure 7-1). First, are the animal data relevant to humans? Animal testing for *developmental* toxicants is generally relevant for human hazard identification (Jelovsek et al., 1989; Francis et al., 1990). While animal data may be less reliable as sources of information about human *reproductive* toxicity, these data have been used successfully to provide presumptive evidence of human reproductive toxicity (NRC, 1989).

Next, it is necessary to determine how to utilize the dose-response information. For example, investigators must consider whether characterization of a benchmark dose, and subsequent calculation of a reference dose, with safety or uncertainty factors, is adequate to protect human health (Barnes and Dourson, 1986; Gaylor, 1989; Kimmel, 1990; Gaylor, 1991). Alternative interpretations must also be considered: in some cases, it may be more appropriate to assume a linear, nonthreshold, low-dose relationship

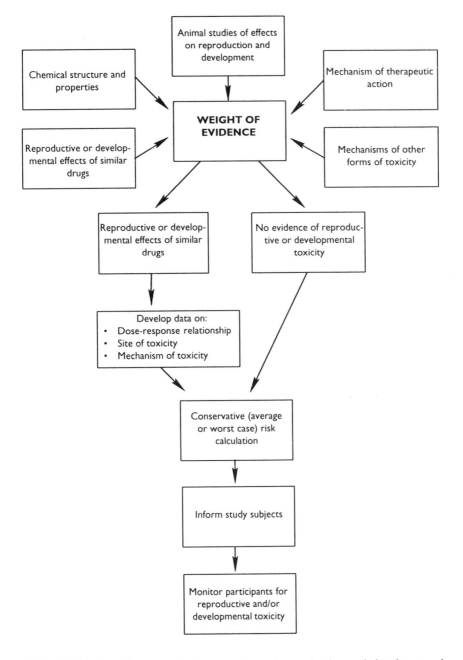

FIGURE 7-1 Considerations in the protection of reproductive and developmental health of research subjects.

between the chemical and the reproductive or developmental effect (Meistrich and Brown, 1983; Rai and Van Ryzin, 1985; Kimmel and Gaylor, 1988; Meistrich, 1989a,b; Kimmel, 1990; Mattison, 1991; Meistrich and Mattison, in press).

Information from animal reproductive tests can be supplemented by other information. For example, data on the nonreproductive toxicity of an agent often provides clues about possible reproductive effects. If an agent is known to be toxic to the nervous system in adults, investigators testing this agent in pregnant animals know to examine the offspring for behavioral function as well as for gross birth defects. Investigators may also utilize what is known about the reproductive effects of certain agents to postulate the effects of related chemicals.

In the rare situation when there is no information on the reproductive and developmental effects of the drug being tested, other approaches may be taken to protect the health of the subject. For example, data from in vitro testing or structure-activity relationships may provide useful information for counseling subjects in a clinical trial. Recent data using expert systems to explore the relationship between chemical structure and developmental toxicity suggest that a substantial amount of useful information could be extracted from existing developmental toxicity data sets (Takihi et al., in press).

Finally, when available, human data on similar agents or classes of agents can be coupled with animal data to develop an overall assessment of an agent's potential for toxicity. In the case of fluoxetine, an antidepressant, the manufacturer collected several hundred cases of exposed pregnancies in which use of the drug was not associated with an increase in birth defects. This sort of evidence is reassuring, but by no means conclusive—an increase in birth defects of the kind and magnitude associated with, for example, valproic acid might not be detected with this number of patients. Arguments for the safety of fluoxetine for use in pregnant women are further strengthened, however, by the observation that rats and rabbits do not show an increase in developmental anomalies when exposed to the drug during pregnancy in standard protocols.

## Subjects' Understanding of Developmental and Reproductive Risks

If men and women of reproductive potential are included in a trial in which they will be exposed to a potential reproductive or developmental toxicant, the potential risks must be characterized as accurately as possible so they can make an informed decision about whether or not to participate. If they decide to participate, they may also wish to consider measures to prevent pregnancy (see below). Finally, information about toxicity risk can help participants determine the likelihood that the baseline incidence of adverse pregnancy outcome will have been increased by study participation, should a pregnancy occur during the trial.

In this regard, the use of reproductive and developmental toxicity information is similar to the use of information about toxicity to other organs and organ systems. Just as investigational agents can be evaluated in preclinical test phases for reproductive and developmental effects, they can be evaluated for carcinogenicity and for toxicity to liver, kidney, and bone marrow. Results from these evaluations are incorporated into the informed consent process, just as reproductive and developmental toxicity information is incorporated.

### Contraception in Clinical Trials

When considering participation in clinical trials of agents with potential reproductive or developmental toxicity, men and women of reproductive age need to be made aware of the contraceptive options available to them as study participants and of what is known about the effectiveness of each method. Table 7-3 lists low and high reported failure rates for the range of contraceptive methods currently available in this country.

The investigator must be concerned with contraception for two major reasons. First, hormonal contraceptives, widely used by women in this country, may introduce complexities into the evaluation of drug effects (see Chapter 4). Second, demographic characteristics of a population can play a role in contraceptive use by that population, with implications for recruitment and the informed consent process.

An investigator may have difficulty assessing the independent effect of a drug in a woman who is using hormonal contraceptives, which can alter the pharmacokinetics (absorption, distribution, metabolism, and excretion) or pharmacodynamics (mechanism of action) of the drug under study. Accurate evaluation of drug effects can also be complicated by the need to clearly isolate the specific side effects of the hormonal contraceptive from those of the drug under study. Where scientific validity or contraceptive effectiveness may be compromised, investigators might consider excluding women using hormonal contraceptives, or recommending that an alternate, nonhormonal method of contraception be used.

There are important differences among population subgroups in the use of contraception, and contraceptive failure rates tend to vary according to age, education, race, ethnicity, marital status, and socioeconomic status. For example, with increasing age, contraceptive failure rates decline as a result of decreased frequency of intercourse and decreased ability to conceive. Non-use of contraceptives is higher among the unmarried, poor, and less educated—a phenomenon that may be associated with access to contraceptive services (Planned Parenthood Federation of America, 1991). Cultural

TABLE 7-3 Methods of Contraception

| Category | Method | Mechanism of Action | Failure Rate[a] Low | High |
|---|---|---|---|---|
| Nonhormonal | No method | | 85.0 | 85.0 |
| | Spermicide alone | Inactivation of sperm | 21.6 | 25.6 |
| | Sponge with spermicide | Mechanical barrier to sperm; inactivation of sperm | 16.0 | 51.9 |
| | Withdrawal | | 14.7 | 27.8 |
| | Periodic abstinence | Avoidance of coitus during presumed fertile days | 13.8 | 19.2 |
| | Diaphragm or cervical cap with spermicide | Mechanical barrier to sperm; inactivation of sperm | 12.0 | 38.9 |
| | Condom | Mechanical barrier to sperm | 9.8 | 18.5 |
| | Intrauterine device, Copper T-380A | Inhibition of sperm migration, fertilization, or ovum transport | 2.5 | 4.5 |
| Hormonal | Oral contraceptives | | 3.8 | 8.7 |
| | Combined | Suppression of ovulation, changes in cervical mucus and endometrium | | |
| | Progestin only | Changes in cervical mucus and endometrium, possibly suppression of ovulation | | |
| | Intrauterine device Progesterone T | Inhibition of sperm migration, fertilization, or ovum transport | 2.5 | 4.5 |
| | Medroxyprogesterone acetate (Depo-Provera) | Changes in cervical mucus and endometrium, suppression of ovulation | <1 | <1 |
| | Levonorgestrel subdermal implants (Norplant) | Same as medroxy-progesterone acetate | <1 | <1 |

[a]Percentage of accidental pregnancies during first year of use. "Low" and "high" refer to rates among women in the United States who were more and less likely than average to use the method correctly and consistently (Harlap, 1991).

and religious norms may also affect some subjects' willingness to use certain forms of contraception. Awareness of these subgroup differences has important implications for both recruitment and informed consent procedures; investigators may wish to modify protocols according to the demographic characteristics of the population to be studied.

## Evaluating Drugs for Use in Lactating Women

Investigators must be especially concerned about developmental toxicity when testing drugs in the subset of the population of reproductive age that is composed of lactating women. Exposure to drugs and chemicals can lead to the presence of these agents in their breast milk, creating concern for: (1) exposure of the infant to the agent and (2) impact of the agent on the quantity and quality of breast milk. Partly as a result of these concerns, lactating women are rarely recruited into trials of new drugs. Therefore, when lactating women require treatment for a medical condition such as pain, infection, depression, constipation, or vitamin deficiency, they often must take medications that have not been systematically evaluated in lactating women. To avoid risk by ceasing lactation during treatment is in many cases not advisable, considering lactation's important benefits (e.g., maternal-infant bonding; transmission to the infant of antibacterial and antiviral substances; enhanced nutrition, growth, and development of the infant).

Factors influencing the presence and amount of a drug in breast milk include maternal and mammary physiology and pharmacokinetics, chemical properties (e.g., lipid solubility, and protein binding), and infant feeding characteristics (frequency, duration, and amount). The impact, if any, of a drug on the child will depend on the amount of drug ingested, the pharmacokinetics of the drug (absorption, distribution, metabolism, and elimination), and the mechanism of action and toxicity of the drug. Not all drugs on the market have been fully characterized for their presence in breast milk and effect on the nursing infant, but some data are available to guide the practitioner; most drugs are compatible with breastfeeding (Briggs et al., 1986). Less well studied is the impact of drugs on milk production. Drugs suspected to alter milk production include dopaminergic agents, estrogen-containing oral contraceptives and other estrogens, antiestrogens, nicotine, prostaglandins, and the thiazide diuretics.

Investigators designing clinical studies in which lactating women may be recruited should carefully advise these women of the risks to the nursing child, including those of or cessation of lactation. Where possible, efforts should be made to characterize risks to the nursing infant based on known pharmacologic and toxicologic properties of an agent in other populations.

## Evaluating Drugs for Use in Pregnant Women

Studies have shown that an average of 3.8 medications are used during each pregnancy (Heinonen et al., 1983) and that 75 percent of pregnant women use between 3 and 10 drugs while they are pregnant (Quirk, 1986). Medications used most commonly during pregnancy include analgesics, antipyretics, antimicrobials, antiemetics, diuretics, cough medications, and psychoactive agents (Quirk, 1986). Yet despite their frequent need for medical treatment, few clinical trials of new drugs include pregnant women. Thus, the initial use of treatments in pregnant women often involves therapies developed in men (and women) who are physiologically different (see Chapter 4).

For clinical conditions that are sufficiently common, controlled trials may be conducted in pregnant women several years after a drug has been put on the market (and several years after pregnant women have been taking the drug on what amounts to an experimental basis). This was true for antihypertensive medications, a number of which were only recently tested in controlled trials for use in pregnancy-induced hypertension. It is not uncommon for physicians to prescribe drugs for pregnant women on the basis of substantial anecdotal information about such use, but reliance on information is risky given the number of cases necessary to identify an association between a drug and an adverse effect.

The testing of therapies in pregnant women often depends on the initiative of independent investigators rather than on the marketing intentions of pharmaceutical manufacturers. It is unusual for a drug to be brought to market for the express purpose of treating pregnancy conditions or pregnant women. An exception is ritodrine, an agent used to treat preterm labor, and which has been marketed expressly for this indication. Ironically, many practitioners use terbutaline or magnesium sulfate to stop preterm labor, although they have not received FDA indications for this purpose. In general, the indications for use restrict the way the drug can be marketed but not how a physician uses the drug. These agents and others (e.g., indomethacin, sulindac, nifedipine) have been tested in controlled trials of preterm labor, although these trials were not part of the drug development efforts for these compounds.

**The committee recommends that NIH strongly encourage and facilitate clinical research to advance the medical management of pre-existing medical conditions in women who become pregnant (e.g., lupus), medical conditions of pregnancy (e.g., gestational diabetes) and, conditions that threaten the successful course of pregnancy (e.g., pre-term labor).**

While the inclusion of pregnant women in clinical studies introduces new complications and risks, the dearth of proven-safe treatment options for ill pregnant women carries its own set of complications and risks. If a drug is going to be used in pregnant women, then the availability of safety and effectiveness information applicable to that population is critical. Reliance upon adverse event reporting by clinicians is not in and of itself a sufficient basis upon which to assess the safety and effectiveness of drugs in pregnant women. Clinical trials, however, also have limitations. Clinical trials have limited power to detect some adverse effects due to the relatively small numbers of subjects included in clinical trials compared with the number of persons who may eventually use the drug under study. Adverse effects may not become evident until the drug is in widespread use. Therefore, systematic surveillance for developmental effects is essential to any plan to include pregnant women in clinical trials. Together, both methods will further our understanding of the medical management of the ill pregnant woman.

## Surveillance for Developmental Effects

Surveillance for reproductive and developmental effects in the offspring is essential to our understanding of the safety of drug use during pregnancy. Such screening assumes that there are tools available to identify developmental effects and that these tools can be economically applied for the surveillance of a healthy population. Procedures may be as simple as a clinical evaluation of the newborn to determine if the child has a structural birth defect that can be identified on physical examination. One of the most critical steps in surveillance is the recording of screening results in a database so that they can be combined with other results for a more comprehensive analysis. Several programs currently exist to monitor populations for congenital malformations; these programs may provide a starting point for surveillance efforts related to pregnant women in clinical studies.

Monitoring of populations for congenital malformations began in the mid-1960s, and by the mid-1970s 7 countries had nationwide monitoring systems and 12 other countries had regional monitoring systems. In addition, the International Clearinghouse for Birth Defects Monitoring was created in the mid-1970s to collect, collate, analyze, and share information on local trends in birth defects identified by the various participating programs; at present there are 26 participating programs.

Monitoring systems use one of two major monitoring strategies: (1) monitoring of all malformations as reported or (2) monitoring of selected "sentinel" malformations, so-called because they are generally detected within the first week of life. Examples of sentinel malformations include anencephaly, spina bifida, hydrocephaly, orofacial clefts, gastrointestinal atresia, deformities of the extremities, Down's syndrome, and congenital hip dislocation. Unfortunately, neither approach escapes the difficulty of ascertainment. Studies indicate that monitoring systems for congenital malformation experience substantial underreporting; in some cases, only one-third of infants with a given abnormality are identified by a monitoring system.

Most monitoring systems have established specific thresholds of malformation incidence that signal a significant increase in frequency (Holtzman and Khoury, 1986). These thresholds are characterized as excesses above an expected number (assumed to be a Poisson variable), excesses above a baseline rate determined from historical information, a decreasing time interval between consecutive births with the malformation (also determined from historical information), or changes in time-space clustering. As in all statistical analysis, it is important to avoid the erroneous assumption of causation when drugs are associated with birth defects. Given the large number of comparisons calculated for adverse developmental outcome, however, false positives are a continual problem.

As is the case with individual clinical trials, it is important to understand the capacity of a monitoring system to identify correctly a developmental toxicant, based on the number of births registered with the system. For example, cleft lip occurs in about 1 in every 1,000 births (incidence is 0.001). The ability to identify an exposure that increases the incidence of cleft lip varies with the size of the population monitored. If 75,000 births are monitored (half treated and half untreated), an increase of 1.3-fold over background could be identified; however, if 10,000 births are monitored (half treated and half untreated), the minimum increase that could be detected would be a 2.0-fold increase above background. In a related sense, the power of monitoring systems to detect adverse effects is also limited because few pregnant women will be exposed to a specific drug. While surveillance cannot guarantee detection of developmental toxicants, systematic collection of information about pregnancy outcomes in a wide range of situations, complemented with information gained through clinical trials that include pregnant women, provides an important element of protection for pregnant women and their offspring.

**The committee recommends that a review be undertaken of existing birth defects monitoring programs to critically define what they are capable of doing and suggest improvements and reasonable expectations for their use.**

Such a review would be of value in the development of reproductive and developmental screening systems and in further consideration of postmarketing surveillance for reproductive and developmental effects.

## ETHICAL ISSUES: RISK-BENEFIT ANALYSIS

Assessing the potential risks and benefits of clinical research is not always an easy task. The very use of phrases such as "risk-benefit equation" and "balancing risks against benefits" has the misleading effect of making it seem that the process enjoys mathematical precision or scientific rigor. The task is made even more difficult because reasonable people disagree both in their evaluations of the magnitude of risks and benefits and how to weigh risks against potential benefits. Different people—be they medical scientists, patients, or healthy volunteers—may value the risks and benefits differently. They may consider some risks worth taking in relation to potential benefits, while other risks may be viewed as unacceptably high in relation to potential benefits.

Assessing risks and potential benefits has both a scientific component and a personal element that varies with the individual making the assessment. By "scientific" we mean that intersubjective agreement can be attained among scientists and researchers based on observations, previous studies, and clinical experience. For example, the identification of the risks and side effects of drugs and the probability of their occurrence is based on experience from earlier studies. Once a sufficiently large population has been studied, medical scientists should be able to agree on what risks might be expected, how likely they are to occur, and their impact on morbidity and mortality. The foregoing sections of this chapter illustrate the scientific dimension of assessing the risks of harm various substances are likely to produce. The same is true of benefits, when benefits are viewed in a relatively narrow, medical sense, best captured by the concept of efficacy: a drug does what it is designed to do—provide a cure, alleviate symptoms, produce a temporary remission, and so on.

But there also is an irreducibly personal element in risk-benefit assessments. By "personal" we mean the insertion of an individual's values, taken in the broadest sense, into the process of assessing the meaning of risks and benefits for one's life or the lives of others, as well as the weighing of risks against benefits. To take a common example, members of IRBs often disagree on how risky a particular procedure actually is.

A committee member who is a member of one IRB reports that heated disputes have arisen over how to characterize the level of risk of lumbar punctures in infants or demented elderly patients, insertion of urethral catheters in six-year-old boys, right-heart catheterization in cardiac patients, withdrawing medication from patients with mild-to-moderate hypertension, and withholding antipsychotic medication from patients with severe emotional disorders. Those who agree on the scientific facts concerning the magnitude and probability of side effects will bring different personal values and experiences to the question of whether the risks are acceptable.

Women's values can differ significantly from those of scientists (whether male or female) in assessing risk-benefit ratios. For example, women's health advocates tend to define the "safety" of contraceptive methods in terms different from those typically employed by biomedical scientists. According to one report:

> Scientists' concern is to establish safety of methods according to specific measurable parameters. They assess toxicity, first in animals and then in carefully controlled studies in human volunteers. Subsequent studies address efficacy and short- to medium-term safety. . . . Women's health advocates . . . give more priority to methods that have fewer side effects and that protect against sexually transmitted diseases and their consequences such as infertility. While scientists have tended to give priority to methods which minimize users' control, women's health advocates prefer methods controlled by the users. [World Health Organization, 1991:11.]

New policies to encourage the inclusion of women, and in particular women of childbearing age, in clinical studies evidence a greater acknowledgment of individual values and a respect of individual autonomy (see, for example, Merkatz et al., 1993). These policies will affect the responsibilities of IRBs and potential participants. The changes will be most evident in the communication of risks to participants and in IRB risk-benefit assessments.

As with any potential participant, a thorough discussion of the risks and potential benefits of participation is a prerequisite for an individual's ability to make an informed decision to enroll in a clinical study. For men and women of reproductive age, reproductive issues affect the type of information included in the informed consent process.

It will be the IRBs' obligation, as with all research involving presumptively competent adults, to continue to ensure that: (1) the selection of potential participants is fair; (2) the informed consent process is adequate; and (3) the risks to participants are outweighed by the potential benefits. This first duty—fair selection—is the subject of the committee's report and thus requires no additional comment. The other two duties will be discussed below.

### Women (Not Pregnant or Lactating) and Men of Reproductive Age

Significant changes have occurred during the committee's tenure, in policies that govern the inclusion of women of childbearing potential in clinical studies, particularly studies of FDA-regulated products (see Chapter 6). FDA issued new guidelines permitting the participation of women of childbearing potential in the early phases of drug trials, and offered three reasons for this decision: (1) scientific gains in study design related to the early identification of gender differences in trials; (2) the ability to reduce the risk of fetal exposure through protocol design; and (3) recent social changes indicating respect for women's autonomy and decisionmaking capacity in reproductive issues. NIH guidelines are currently under revision. These policy changes should have the effect of including more women of reproductive age in clinical studies, with implications for risk-benefit assessments.

In a study that poses risks to potential offspring, women who are not pregnant at the outset of the investigation may become pregnant while they are still participants. The committee believes that the informed consent process for these women should include information about contraception and the alternatives of voluntarily withdrawing from the study and terminating a pregnancy should conception take place. Similar discussions should be held with men who could father a child while participating in the study. As in all research involving human participants, every effort should be made to ensure that the consent decision is fully voluntary. An example of language for consent forms proposed by Moreno (1994) in his presentation to the committee appears below, as modified by the committee:

> It is possible that your participation in this study may cause damage to children if you choose to have them. You have already been told what is known about this possibility, and you are encouraged to ask further questions. (Include as appropriate: We urge you or your partner not to become pregnant while you are part of this study.) You may want to discuss this with others before you agree to take part in this study. If you wish, we will arrange for a doctor, nurse or counselor who is not part of this study to discuss this possibility with you and anyone else you want to have present.

**The committee recommends that investigators and IRBs not exclude persons of reproductive age from participation in clinical studies. In the case of women of reproductive age, the potential or prospect of becoming pregnant during the study may not be used as a justification for precluding or limiting participation. Risks to the reproductive system should be considered in the same manner as risks to other organ systems. Risks to possible offspring of both men and women who are not pregnant or lactating should not be considered in the risk-benefit calculation. It is the responsibility of investigators and IRBs to assure that the informed consent process include an adequate discussion of risks to reproduction and potential offspring, including, where appropriate, an adequate discussion of relevant considerations of birth control.**

**The committee recommends that the participant be permitted to select voluntarily the contraceptive method of his or her choice where there are no relevant study-dependent, scientific reasons to require**

the exclusion of use of certain contraceptives (e.g., drug interaction).

**The committee recommends that pregnancy termination options be discussed as part of the consent process in clinical studies that pose unknown or foreseeable risks to potential offspring.**

### Lactating Women

The possible transmission of drugs to nursing infants is a risk that must be considered when including lactating women in clinical studies. This additional consideration must be thoroughly discussed in the informed consent process.

**The committee recommends that investigators and IRBs not exclude women who are lactating from participation in clinical studies. It is the responsibility of investigators and IRBs to ensure that the informed consent process includes, wherever appropriate, an advisory to potential participants that there may be special risks to their children if nursing mothers participate. No nursing mother should be permitted to agree to participate without first receiving additional information about these special risks.**

### Pregnant Women

As reflected in the recommendation presented earlier in this chapter, the committee wishes to encourage clinical research to advance the medical management of pregnant women who are or may become ill. In this context, the committee reviewed the current DHHS regulations concerning the involvement of pregnant women as research subjects. The committee's review was limited to situations in which the pregnant woman is the subject of the research (see Chapter 6). It did *not* include situations in which the fetus is the subject of the research (currently covered by the same regulation); fetal research was outside of the committee's charge.

The DHHS regulations begin with a presumption of exclusion—that is, "no pregnant woman may be a research subject" except under certain conditions. The regulations also require that IRBs ensure during their review of research protocols that the exclusionary standard enunciated in the regulations is met. In addition, the regulations classify pregnant women as a "vulnerable population" deserving of special protection. For the reasons discussed below, the committee concluded that the current regulatory scheme should be revised.

The committee acknowledges that the current regulations (45 C.F.R. 46

Subpart B) may reflect an inadvertent attribution of the vulnerability of the fetus (which obviously lacks autonomy) to the pregnant woman. Nonetheless, it is inappropriate for the regulations to retain a presumption of exclusion on the basis that pregnant women are a "vulnerable population" in need of special protection. In this context, "vulnerable" suggests that pregnant women are less autonomous or more easily exploited than other persons—an inference that the committee has found no evidence to support. The labeling of pregnant women as a vulnerable population also might be viewed as suggesting that they cannot weigh the risks to a fetus or potential child in deciding whether to enroll in a clinical study; that pregnant women do not care sufficiently about the health or well-being of their future children to make sound decisions; and that the prevention of all potentially harmful outcomes of pregnancy is a goal that warrants governmental, regulatory, or other official intervention into the lives and free choices of women. The committee rejects these inferences as well. Removal of pregnant women from the regulatory category of "vulnerable" potential subjects would avoid any possible inference that pregnant women are less capable of making informed decisions by virtue of their pregnancy, than are other potential research participants.

For all potential research participants, risk-benefit assessment is a complex and difficult task. Nevertheless, it is no more difficult for pregnant women than it is for nonpregnant women or for men. Virtually all women desire healthy infants, even when their pregnancies are unplanned. While occasionally there may be pregnant women who are incapable of acting in the interests of their future children, it would be inappropriate to base a public policy on an atypical case, rather than a normative case.

There also is little public support for the proposition that the prevention of all potentially harmful outcomes of pregnancy is a goal that warrants governmental, regulatory, or other official intervention into the lives and free choices of women. Pregnant women may choose to work in stressful jobs, engage in recreational activities, drive automobiles, and do other things that could place their own or their fetuses' health or life in jeopardy.

**The committee recommends that pregnant women be presumed to be eligible for participation in clinical studies. It is the responsibility of investigators and IRBs to ensure that pregnant women are provided with adequate information about the risks and benefits to themselves, their pregnancies and their potential offspring. Even when evidence concerning risks is unknown or ambiguous,[1] the decision about acceptability of risk to the pregnancy or to offspring should be made by the woman as part of the informed consent process.**

The committee was unanimous in the view that pregnant women should be presumed to be eligible for participation in clinical studies. The committee also unanimously endorsed the importance of recognizing, in public policy as well as in the deliberations of IRBs and investigators, that pregnant women should be treated as competent adults capable of making their own decisions about participation in research. It should be emphasized that the committee is not recommending that NIH impose an affirmative obligation on investigators to recruit pregnant women into every clinical study. What follows is further explication of the committee's intent with respect to the implementation of this recommendation.

## Adequate Information

With respect to the obligation to ensure that pregnant women are provided with adequate information about the risks and benefits to their pregnancy and potential offspring, the committee recommends the following strengthened informed consent procedure. The disclosure statement of consent forms for all studies that pose a risk to pregnancy or potential offspring should include, highlighted in bold type, a statement such as: *If you are pregnant or contemplating pregnancy, we urge you to consult your obstetrical care provider before deciding about participation in this study. Participation in this study may (does) pose a risk of (significant) harm to your pregnancy and/or your potential baby.*

Investigators should ask all potential participants if they are pregnant as part of the initial screening phase of recruitment. If a woman is pregnant, her attention should be drawn to this bolded statement. This process should include a special disclosure statement that details in easily understood lay language what is known about the risks and potential benefits to her pregnancy and potential offspring, resulting from participation in the study. This statement should be reviewed with the pregnant woman, and she should be encouraged to consult with her obstetrical care provider before proceeding further in the consent process. It is important for a pregnant woman to have benefit of the advice of her obstetrical care provider in deciding whether to participate in a study. (In the case where the woman's own obstetrical care provider is the study investigator, the pregnant woman should be offered the opportunity to discuss her participation with a similarly qualified individual who is not associated with the study.) If the pregnant woman does not wish to consult with her obstetrical care provider, and even if she has had such a consultation, specific procedures should be instituted to ensure that she understands the relevant risks and benefits. For example, the potential participant could be asked to describe in her own words what the risks and benefits are. It should be clear that the pregnant woman understands that no drug or other intervention can improve on normal pregnancy in a healthy woman. Alternatively, the pregnant woman could be asked to complete a knowledge test. Deficiencies in understanding discovered through either method should be addressed through continued discussion and education. Only after the woman demonstrates an adequate understanding should consent be solicited. These are procedures that are generally advocated to improve the quality and the meaningfulness of the informed consent process (Faden and Beauchamp, 1986; Appelbaum et al., 1987). They are particularly important when the stakes associated with participation are high, as is the case for pregnant women if participation entails significant risks to pregnancy or potential offspring.

## Paternal Consent

It is appropriate for investigators to encourage a potential participant who is pregnant to discuss her participation in clinical studies and risks to potential offspring with the potential baby's father, but the committee rejects any requirement that the consent of the potential baby's father be a condition of the participation of a pregnant woman in research. The committee recognizes that the husbands of pregnant women, as well as future fathers who are not husbands, have an interest in the health of their children and that these men may have a deep emotional attachment toward their offspring prior to birth. Until a child is born, however, the future father can only protect the health of the potential child by controlling the decisions and actions of the woman. To give men the authority to veto the decisions of their wives or partners to participate in research grants men unacceptable power over women. It also would accord greater protection to fetuses than to children; only one parent's permission is required to enroll an infant or child in clinical research.

## Scientific Criteria for Exclusion

The committee recognizes that, as in all clinical studies, there may be scientifically and medically valid reasons for excluding pregnant women from a particular study. A pregnant woman would be excluded if the medical condition of pregnancy disqualifies her as a subject in the same sense that anyone else, pregnant or nonpregnant, male or female, would be disqualified based on medical conditions that would interfere scientifically with the study. For example, a pregnant woman would be excluded from a study of hormone replacement or contraception. A pregnant woman also would be excluded from a study of weight loss, as would any person who, for example, was already very underweight; scientifically, it would not make sense to include either type of person in such a study. Similarly, a pregnant woman would be excluded from a study when the condition of pregnancy places the *woman* in a risk category (because pregnancy increases the risk of harm to the woman) that would exclude others due to an unacceptable risk/benefit ratio.

### Other Criteria for Exclusion

There was considerable discussion within the committee about whether there are any exceptional instances in which IRBs can be given the discretion to exclude pregnant women from participation for other than scientific reasons. Most committee members ultimately endorsed the following recommendation:

> **Investigators and IRBs may exclude pregnant women from participation only when the IRB finds, and records its finding in writing, that the following standard has been met: (1) there is no prospect of medical benefit to the pregnant woman, and (2) a risk of significant harm to potential offspring is known or can be plausibly inferred.**

A finding that a risk of significant harm to potential offspring is "known or can be plausibly inferred" may be based on evidence from animal studies, in vitro studies, structure-activity relationship data, or previous clinical experience.

Under this standard, IRBs may exclude pregnant women from the earliest phases of many drug trials, but most clinical studies would remain open to pregnant women. Committee members adopting this standard were motivated by a desire to be true to the underlying principle that pregnant women should be treated no differently than other presumptively competent adults in the context of IRB deliberations. In addition, these committee members were particularly concerned that if the exceptive case was not narrowly constructed, variation in interpretation could open the door to widespread exclusions of pregnant women.

A few members of the committee, however, were not able to endorse the above mentioned standard. They wished to reserve for the IRB the discretion to exclude pregnant women from participation not only when there is no prospect of medical benefit to the women but also when there is only potential for benefit to them that could be characterized as minimal or insignificant. The intent here is to allow the IRB more room for judgment about the appropriateness of exclusion. An example of a situation in which these members believed that IRBs should have the discretion to exclude pregnant women was that of a clinical trial of a medication thought to be helpful in the management of severe acne but known to cause malformations in offspring if taken during pregnancy. The standard endorsed by most committee members would not permit a blanket exclusion of pregnant women from such a study, as it could not be claimed that there is no prospect of medical benefit to the pregnant participant.

The committee also struggled with how to accommodate within its support for the shift of the presumption to *inclusion* of pregnant women (from that of exclusion) a role for conscience and an individual investigator's moral commitments. It was agreed that, at a minimum, such a mechanism would require that the investigator provide the IRB with a written explanation of his or her concerns of conscience and that the IRB review any such requests in light of a presumption that favors the inclusion of pregnant women in clinical studies. It also would require the IRB to guard against any abuse of conscience claims, and, in particular, against circumstances in which a request for exemption on the basis of conscience is offered in lieu of other reasons not based in moral commitment. It is precisely because of the potential for abuse of a "conscience" exemption that the committee could not resolve whether or under what conditions such an exemption should be constructed. Appeals to conscience are in many respects unassailable; in some contexts, the force of such appeals has had a chilling effect on public policy.

## Documentation and Monitoring of Exclusions

An IRB must record in writing both its reasons for permitting any exception to the general presumption of inclusion of pregnant women and the frequency with which it grants such exceptions. It is anticipated that IRBs would record such information in the minutes of their meetings and that the act of documentation would help the IRBs to properly implement the standard. Such record keeping also would provide a source of information should OPRR desire to evaluate the performance of an IRB on this issue.

## Conclusion

The committee recognizes that its recommendation concerning the participation of pregnant women in clinical studies cannot ensure the prevention of a small, theoretical risk of harm to offspring. Pregnancy and the controversial moral and legal standing of the fetus or potential child raise unique considerations. We do not wish to dismiss or evade these important considerations. However, the committee was persuaded of the overriding value of ensuring that all women—pregnant or otherwise—be treated justly with respect to the opportunity to derive the benefits of research. The shifting of the presumption to one of *inclusion* of pregnant women in clinical studies from one of *exclusion* is an important step in that direction.

The committee believes that given the safeguards described above, holding IRBs and investigators to the presumption of including pregnant women in research is not a significant threat to the health of future generations. Except for studies specifically designed to investigate outcomes in pregnant women—which the committee strongly endorses—it is exceedingly unlikely that investigators will seek out pregnant women for recruitment. It should be emphasized that the committee is not recommending that NIH impose an affirmative obligation on investigators to recruit pregnant women into every clinical study. Moreover, the committee's conclusions are consistent with the position that women who are or who might become pregnant have a moral obligation to weigh risks to a future child when deciding whether to participate as research subjects. It is unlikely that pregnant women will seek admission into studies that pose a significant risk of harm to their offspring, unless there is some offsetting benefit to the health of the pregnant woman that in turn advances the interests of the potential child by its having a healthy mother. A policy of presuming that pregnant women are eligible to participate in clinical research, although introducing a possibility of harm to a potential child, is in fact likely to produce health dividends for mothers that will inure to their children. Although the committee is not indifferent to the risk of harm to even one potential child, the committee felt compelled to consider as primary the interests of all women in being treated justly and with dignity.

**The committee recommends that OPRR revise and reissue Subpart B of the DHHS regulations for the Protection of Human Subjects, titled "Additional Protections Pertaining to Research, Development, and Related Activities Involving Fetuses, Pregnant Women, and Human In-vitro Fertilization [45 C.F.R. 46, subpart B] in accordance with the committee's recommendations.**

At least a technical amendment to Subpart A, sec. 46.111(a)(3), eliminating the reference to pregnant women as a "vulnerable population" will be required by this revision to Subpart B.

## NOTE

1. There is historical precedent for classification of unknown or ambiguous risks to the fetus as more than minimal. This policy was developed with respect to fetoscopy in a decision by the Department of Health, Education, and Welfare Ethics Advisory Board in 1979 (DHEW, 1979) and by the NIH with respect to chorion villi sampling in the 1980s (C. McCarthy, former director of NIH Office of Protection from Research Risks, personal communication, October 1993). In both cases, it proved to be an appropriate

presumption, since both procedures were subsequently determined to increase the risk of spontaneous abortion. IRBs and investigators may find it helpful to use this convention in discussing the level of risk with potential participants.

## REFERENCES

Appelbaum, P.S., Roth, L.H., Lidz, C.W., Benson, P., and Winslade, W. 1987. False hopes and best data: Consent to research and the therapeutic misconception. *Hastings Center Report* 17(April):20-24.

Barnes, D.G., and Dourson, M. 1986. Reference dose (RfD): Description and use in health risk assessments. *Regulatory Toxicology Pharmacology* 8:471-486.

Briggs, G.G., Freeman, R.K., and Yaffe, F.J. 1986. Drugs in Pregnancy and Lactation: A Reference Guide to Fetal and Neonatal Risk. 2nd ed. Baltimore, Md.: Williams & Wilkins.

DHEW (Department of Health, Education, and Welfare). 1979. DHEW Support of Fetoscopy. Report and Recommendations of the DHEW Secretary's Ethics Advisory Board, 23 February.

Faden, R.R., and Beauchamp, T.L. 1986. *A History and Theory of Informed Consent*. New York: Oxford University Press.

Fletcher, J.C., and Ryan, K.J. Federal regulations for fetal research: A case for reform. *Law, Medicine and Health Care* 15(3):126-138.

Francis, E.Z., Kimmel, C.A., and Rees, D.C. 1990. Workshop on the qualitative and quantitative comparability of human and animal developmental neurotoxicity: Summary and implications. *Neurotoxicology and Teratology* 12(3):285-292.

Gaylor, D.W. 1991. Comparison of the properties of reference doses based on the NOAEL and benchmark doses. *Proceedings, Air and Waste Management Association* 71: paper no. 91-173.6.

Gaylor, D.W. 1989. Quantitative risk analysis for quantal reproductive and developmental effects. *Environmental Health Perspectives* 79:243-246.

Harlap, S. 1991. Preventing pregnancy, protecting health. New York: Alan Guttmacher Institute.

Heinonen, O.P., Sloan, E.D., and Shapiro, S. 1983. Birth Defects and Drugs in Pregnancy. Boston: John Wright.

Holtzman, N.A., and Khoury, M.J. 1986. Monitoring for congenital malformations. *Annual Review of Public Health* 7:237-266.

Jelovsek, F.R., Mattison, D.R., and Chen, J.J. 1989. Prediction of risk for human developmental toxicity: How important are animal studies for hazard identification? *Obstetrics and Gynecology* 74:624-635.

Jelovsek, F.R., Mattison, D.R., and Young, J.F. 1990. Eliciting principles of hazard identification from experts. *Teratology* 42:521-533.

Kimmel, C.A. 1990. Quantitative approaches to human risk assessment for noncancer health effects. *Neurotoxicology* 11:189-198.

Kimmel, C.A., and Gaylor, D.W. 1988. Issues and qualitative and quantitative risk analysis for developmental toxicology. *Risk Analysis* 8:15-20.

Kline, J., Stein, Z., and Susser, M. 1989. Conception to Birth: Epidemiology of Prenatal Development. New York: Oxford University Press.

Koren, G., Bologna, M., and Pastyszak, A. 1990. The way women perceive teratogenic risk: The decision to terminate pregnancy. Pp. 373-381 in Maternal-Fetal Toxicology: A Clinician's Guide, G. Koren, ed. New York: Marcel Dekker.

Koren, G., Bologna, M., Long, D., Feldman, Y., and Shear, N.H. 1989. Perception of teratogenic risk by pregnant women exposed to drugs and chemicals during the first trimester. *American Journal of Obstetrics and Gynecology* 160:1190-1194.

Mattison, D.R. 1991. An overview of biological markers in reproductive and developmental toxicology: Concepts, definitions and use in risk assessment. *Biomedical and Environmental Sciences* 4:8-34.

Merkatz, R., Temple, R., Sobel, S., Feiden, K., Kessler, D., and the Working Group on Women in Clinical Trials. 1993. *New England Journal of Medicine* 329(4):292-296.

Meistrich, M. 1989a. Calculations of the incidence of infertility in human populations from sperm measures using the two-distribution model. Pp. 275-290 in Institute for Health Policy Analysis Forum on Science, Health, and Environmental Risk Assessment. Alan R. Liss.

Meistrich, M. 1989b. Interspecies comparison and quantitative extrapolation of toxicity to the human male reproductive system. In Toxicology of the Male and Female Reproductive Systems, P.K. Working, ed. Bristol, Penn.: Hemisphere.

Meistrich, M., and Brown, C.C. 1983. Estimation of the increased risk of human infertility from alterations in semen characteristics. *Fertility and Sterility* 40(2):220-230.

Meistrich, M., and Mattison, D.R. In press. Methods for quantitative assessment of reproductive risks. In: Assessing the Risks of Adverse Reproductive Outcomes, Monograph No. 4 of the Conte Institute for Environmental Health, D. Brenner and A. Bloom, eds. March of Dimes.

Moreno, J.D. 1994. Ethical issues related to the inclusion of women of childbearing potential in clinical trials. In: Women and Health Research: Ethical and Legal Issues of Including Women in Clinical Studies, Volume 2, A. Mastroianni, R. Faden, and D. Federman, eds. Washington, D.C.: National Academy Press.

NRC (National Research Council) 1983. Risk Assessment in the Federal Government: Managing the Process. Washington, D.C.: National Academy Press.

NRC. 1989. Biologic Markers in Reproductive Toxicology. Washington, D.C.: National Academy Press.

Olshein, A.R., and Mattison, D.R., eds. In press. Male Mediated Developmental Toxicity. New York: Plenum.

Phelan, M.C., Pelloch, J.M., and Nance, W.E. 1982. Discordant expression of fetal hydantoin syndrome in heteropaternal twins. *New England Journal of Medicine* 307:99-101.

Planned Parenthood Federation of America. 1991. New Birth Control Conferences Report. Nine Conferences in Nine Cities: A Report, January 1990-January 1991. New York: Planned Parenthood Federation of America.

Quirk, J.G. 1986. Use and misuse of drugs in pregnancy. In: Drug and Chemical Action in Pregnancy: Pharmacologic and Toxicologic Principles, S. Fabro and A.R. Scialli, eds. New York: Marcel Dekker.

Rai, K., and Van Ryzin, J. 1985. A dose response model for teratological experiments involving quantal responses. *Biometrics* 41:1-9.

Schardein, J.L. 1985. Chemically Induced Birth Defects. New York: Marcel Dekker.

Shepard, T.H. 1983. Catalog of Teratogenic Agents, 4th ed. Baltimore, Md.: Johns Hopkins University Press.

Sherwin, S. 1992. No Longer Patient. Philadelphia: Temple University Press.

Takihi, N., Rosenkranz, H.S., Klopman, G., and Mattison, D.R. In press. Structural determinants of developmental toxicity. Submitted to the Conference Proceedings for Workshop on Quantitative Methods in Developmental Toxicology, National Research Council, Washington, D.C.

Wilson, J.G., and Fraser, F.C., eds. 1979. Handbook of Teratology. New York: Plenum.

World Health Organization Special Programme of Research, Development and Research Training in Human Reproduction and International Women's Health Coalition. 1991. Creating Common Ground: Women's Perspectives on the Selection and Introduction of Fertility Regulation Technologies. Geneva: World Health Organization.

Zar, J.H. 1984. Biostatistical Analysis. Englewood Cliffs, N.J.: Prentice-Hall.

# 8

# Implementation

Policies requiring the inclusion of women and racial and ethnic groups in clinical studies are already in place. These policies are proactive in that they seek to bring the conduct of clinical studies into line with some general principles of inclusion of diverse population groups as research subjects. The policies assume that the current activities of publicly and privately funded scientists can be viewed as a collective national research enterprise in which there is mutual accountability for the overall extent to which various health problems and population groups are studied. These policies also assume (but do not assure) that processes can be established whereby the desired level of inclusiveness will be achieved. By bringing the force of law to bear upon the research enterprise, the authors of these mandates— Congress, the National Institutes of Health (NIH), and the Food and Drug Administration (FDA)—also imply that the desired levels of inclusiveness do not now exist and would probably not develop spontaneously.

The present emphasis placed by NIH on the recruitment of diverse population groups into clinical research is a strong initial step in the pursuit of equity in clinical studies. Where earlier versions of the current NIH policy on inclusion of women in clinical studies simply encouraged investigators to include women in study populations, more recent policy statements require that "clear and compelling" rationales be given for the exclusion of women from proposed studies. More important, efforts to disseminate the policy statement to investigators and reviewers have been bolstered. NIH has conducted a review of the impact of the revised (1991) policy and, while the results are not yet available, it is expected that the level of women's participation in clinical studies will be significant.

The challenge for those involved in clinical research is how to achieve full implementation of these policies in a way that enhances the overall research enterprise, while simultaneously dealing with the apparent theoretical, methodological, and regulatory complications they pose for investigators, sponsors, peer review and regulatory bodies, and research participants. Of particular relevance to this report is the challenge of anticipating and resolving the social, ethical, and legal dilemmas that may arise in the attempt to achieve equity in our pluralistic society. For example, both the revised guidelines from NIH on the inclusion of subpopulations in research studies and the provisions of the NIH Revitalization Act of 1993 (the "Act") requiring that each NIH-funded study include representative samples of subpopulations unless their absence is justified, have caused concern among many people, including the members of this committee, about the feasibility and cost of conducting clinical studies in accordance with these new mandates.

An important consequence of implementing the demands of justice in the context of clinical research is the improvement of scientific knowledge and the ability to address the health problems of *all* peoples. The Act clearly is intended to promote this goal by changing the prevailing presumption to one of inclusion. The Act requires investigators to both justify any gender or racial or ethnic exclusions and identify and analyze gender differences. The committee fully endorses the spirit of these requirements. Investigators should be obligated to be inclusive in their recruitment practices and to justify any departure in the composition of their study populations from what might be expected given the characteristics of the problem under investigation. The committee is concerned, however, that if the act is too rigidly interpreted, it will make costly and undue demands on the scientific research process and impede the implementation of its noble goal. The committee has offered specific recommendations intended to ensure that questions of justice and inclusion are a top priority at every level of the research process. The committee does not believe that the interests of justice in advancing the health of all people are best served by a requirement that *every* clinical trial be large enough to conduct valid analyses of every relevant subgroup comparison. As reflected in the committee's guiding principles 1 and 2, (see Chapter 3), the ultimate burden for achieving justice falls on the national research agenda as a whole and cannot be implemented by a mechanical approach to the selection of subjects on a study-by-study basis.

The preceding chapters have laid out the rationale and guiding principles for including greater numbers of women in clinical studies; they also identified the considerations—ethical, scientific, social, and legal—that might impede the achievement of this goal. In the process of presenting this material, the committee has stated a number of its conclusions and recommendations with regard to the broad shape and general direction of this process. In this final chapter, many of these broad recommendations are tied to the specific actors and actions needed to achieve a collective national research effort that—in both practice and perception—will equitably address the health concerns of the diverse populations that make up our society. Some of these actions involve short-term strategies that can be implemented almost immediately; others involve the strengthening of existing mechanisms or institutions; still others depend upon processes that do not yet exist and may take considerable time to establish.

The overall long-term goal of these activities is to improve our scientific knowledge and ability to address the health problems of all peoples. The committee believes that this will require the active involvement of all sectors of the research community. While these recommendations concentrate on the NIH research structure, the committee also recognizes the vital contributions of pharmaceutical companies and other nonfederal sponsors to the overall research enterprise. Therefore, the committee recommends that the spirit of the recommendations in this chapter be appropriately modified and applied by private and nonprofit sponsors in their research context. Furthermore, enhanced efforts to coordinate federal, private, and nonprofit research efforts are encouraged.

The committee believes that everyone involved in the conduct of research—project investigators, institutional review boards (IRBs), initial review groups (IRGs), technical evaluation groups (TEGs) (together, IRGs and TEGs are commonly known as study sections), scientific advisory councils, and NIH management—must participate in this process. Therefore, while the recommendations are made to NIH, they specifically address each step in the process, from the conception of the research project by the investigator, to the review process of IRBs, to the scientific review boards, IRGs and TEGs (study sections), the implementation of the overall research agenda by the NIH advisory councils, and finally to the overall assurance of accomplishing the research mission by NIH.

The ultimate criteria for judging the success of a public policy to achieve justice and promote inclusion will be changes in research policy and clinical practice, and ultimately improvements in health status indicators, particularly in areas where unjustifiable disparities currently exist. Specific objectives include the following:

• Establish accountability for implementation at every level of the research enterprise, including levels well above that of the individual investigator;
• Provide the necessary database to shape adherence and identify gaps in knowledge;

• Establish a system for monitoring compliance with specific inclusion-based requirements and evaluating the extent to which fairness is being achieved;

• Use the preceding processes and data bases to educate, inform, and promote discussion among policy makers, bureaucrats, investigators, IRBs, IRGs, TEGs, and the general public.

## RECOMMENDATIONS

The committee has divided its recommendations into two categories: those that can be implemented immediately and maintained over the long term; and those that will depend on preparatory steps and should be implemented as soon as feasible. Recommendations to address objectives of accountability, for example, can and should be implemented immediately. Recommendations for the development of new databases, however, cannot be fully implemented until consistent changes in data collection have been achieved.

NIH already requires reporting of the composition of study populations, which keeps investigators aware of the need to involve diverse populations. Additional resources, supports, and monitoring strengthen this effort by providing numerous opportunities at each level within the review process for the evaluation, referral, and revision of protocols. The committee strongly endorses the principle that tracking the study population composition and topics of funded studies and providing this information on a regular basis to all those involved in the research process will in and of itself raise the level of awareness and activity concerning the issues of both study composition and attention to women's health concerns. The assessment of accumulated research is the most comprehensive mechanism for monitoring the implementation of the policy of inclusion. The protocol review suggested here, however, increases the likelihood that questionable protocols will be recognized early and handled effectively.

### The Investigator

**Immediate Actions**

The committee believes that tracking both the composition of study populations and topics of funded studies, and providing this information on a regular basis to all those involved in the research process, will, in and of itself, raise the level of awareness and activity concerning the issues of both study composition and attention to women's health concerns. NIH already requires investigators to report the composition of study populations, which keeps investigators aware of the need to involve diverse populations. It is important that individual investigators be aware of both the state of the science and the state of clinical practice with respect to gender and other subgroup differences in their areas of research. **In designing studies, investigators should conduct literature reviews to determine (1) the extent to which an evidentiary base exists for suspecting gender-specific and subgroup effect, and (2) the extent to which women and other groups have served as participants in relevantly similar research.**

**If there is a plausible basis for suspecting gender differences, investigators should make every effort to recruit sufficient participants of both genders to conduct analyses to detect these differences. In the absence of such an evidentiary base, investigators should recruit participants of both genders. Where sample size is large enough, investigators also should conduct analysis of gender differences in these studies.** Investigators should strive to collect sufficient data on gender-related variables to permit a refined interpretation of any observed gender differences (e.g., potential confounders or mechanistic variables such as hormonal status of women, weight, and adiposity) and to reveal trends or suggest hypotheses.

## As Soon as Feasible

**Investigators should draw on the expertise available in the social science community to improve the ways in which the variables of gender, race, and ethnicity are conceptualized, operationalized, and measured in their studies.** Such collegial exchanges will enable investigators to tailor their study designs, recruitment and retention efforts, and informed consent procedures to the study population selected, to avoid unwarranted exclusions of potential participants, and to be prepared to collect sufficient data on gender-related and subgroup variables to analyze for confounding effects.

Investigators clearly need broad-based support from the other actors within the research process in order to carry out their part of a comprehensive agenda. **The committee recommends that IRBs, IRGs, TEGs, scientific advisory councils, and NIH management become more directly involved with investigators in activities that promote development of more inclusive study designs.** Measures recommended by the committee, such as IRB review of protocols for study population composition and NIH provision of opportunities for investigator training and access to needed databases, facilitate investigator efforts to realize the goal of greater inclusion.

## The IRB

### Immediate Actions

As part of the IRBs' responsibility for ensuring the just selection of persons to be participants in research, IRBs should require investigators to provide the proposed gender, racial, and ethnic composition for each study, as well as information about the distribution of the condition under study in the population at large and the composition of subjects in previous relevant research. It is the IRBs' responsibility to make a determination that the composition of the proposed study is equitable.

### As Soon as Feasible

**IRBs, in concert with NIH, should engage in educational efforts that will ensure awareness among investigators of gender and racial and ethnic biases.** Research organizations could draw upon the expertise of social scientists experienced in the conceptualization, operationalization, measurement, and analysis of variables relevant to these issues to assist investigators.

The committee believes that providing feedback to IRBs concerning the characteristics of the study populations and research topics it has approved will serve to raise the level of awareness of IRBs to issues of justice and inclusion. **The NIH Office of Protection from Research Risks (OPRR) should require IRBs to collect data on study population composition and research topics of all studies subject to IRB review.** OPRR could monitor study population composition through, for example, a representative sample of general assurance IRBs.

## IRGs and TEGs

### Immediate Actions

Once NIH policies for inclusion of gender, racial, and ethnic groups are finalized, it is anticipated that IRGs and TEGs will have significant responsibility for monitoring their implementation. As with any new policy, it is expected that in the initial stages of implementation guidance will be needed. **NIH should develop a mechanism for monitoring the actions taken by IRGs and TEGs in implementing policies for inclusion of gender, racial, and ethnic groups, and provide feedback to the IRGs and TEGs in order to ensure consistent and appropriate interpretation of these policies.** Among other tools for evaluation, NIH might consider taking a random sample of justifications for exclusions. Central review and evaluation can standardize the implementation of the policy, and it will correct both unnecessarily strict and overly lenient policy interpretations by the peer review system. It will also provide illustrative material for education of IRG and TEG members as recommended below.

## As Soon as Feasible

**Each IRG and TEG should recruit members with expertise in the area of gender, racial, and ethnic differences or persons sensitive to gender and racial and ethnic concerns. Furthermore, every member of IRGs and TEGs should receive training and education on evaluation of study population composition and gender, racial, and ethnic differences.** The very presence of qualified males and females from different racial and ethnic backgrounds is one way of increasing the likelihood that the relevant questions and appropriate conceptualizations are considered by investigators. A rough measure of sensitivity could be based on professional activities, such as research agenda, participation in committees of professional associations, publications, and service at one's institution.

## Scientific Advisory Councils

### As Soon as Feasible

**Mechanisms should be developed for ensuring that principles of justice are central considerations in the setting of the nation's research agenda.** Because clinical research carries both benefits and burdens, justice requires that no one group—gender, racial, ethnic or socioeconomic—receive disproportionate benefits or bear disproportionate burdens of research. For the overall biomedical research agenda to comply with the requirements of justice, studies must not only include women as well as men, but also women and men from different age cohorts and different racial and ethnic groups. In addition, the health needs of all women and men should receive their fair share of research resources and attention. Scientific advisory councils have the ultimate responsibility for determining priorities in the research agenda for the subject matter area they cover. These decisions should move toward establishing equity in U.S. research efforts for all populations over time. Databases compiled by NIH can be used by scientific advisory councils in making decisions about research priorities within the available funding and in determining what areas require requests for proposals (RFPs) or requests for applications (RFAs) to improve the balance of research across diseases and subgroups. The heads of the councils should confer periodically to assess the application of principles of justice across research areas.

In developing research priorities, these councils should give special consideration as to whether the health needs of pregnant women are being adequately addressed by their institutes.

## NIH

### Immediate Actions

**NIH should maintain the current policy emphasis on the inclusion of women in NIH-supported clinical studies.** NIH should continue the practice of identifying research concerns of various subgroups (gender, race, ethnicity, socioeconomic status) and offer RFAs and RFPs for such studies. **Where new requirements for subgroup analysis result in increases in study size and additional recruitment strategies, supplemental funds (e.g., from the NIH Office of Research on Women's Health) should be made available to meet these funding challenges.**

**NIH should commission studies to determine the present state of scientific knowledge on gender, racial, and ethnic differences to help investigators determine where subgroup analysis would be likely to identify clinically significant differences.** These efforts should culminate in the establishment of a database that includes such information as differences in disease incidence and prevalence, as well as relevant physiological and cultural differences in subgroups. Investigators would be able to consult this database in developing strategies to identify and detect gender, racial, and ethnic differences.

**NIH should require that proposals for clinical studies include in their literature reviews the following: the extent to which an evidentiary base exists for suspecting gender or other subgroup differences relevant to the proposed research; the demographic characteristics of subjects in past similar research; groups for which the proposed study might have special relevance; how the preceding information justifies the population selected for the proposed study; and how that choice will address gaps identified in the literature.** This requirement should be incorporated into the guidelines on the grant application (PHS 398 form).

**NIH should widely disseminate to the scientific community methodological guidance on: (1) compliance with the legislative mandate regarding the inclusion of women and other subgroups in clinical research and (2) considerations for valid subgroup analysis.**

### As Soon as Feasible

**NIH should pursue the current dialogue with Congress and the research community on the policy of inclusion and the commitment to justice.** The objective is to develop mechanisms that merge public policy goals with scientific advice to promote legislation that is at once socially responsible, practical, and consistent with good science. Such action would extract the scientific community from a current dilemma: if NIH is strictly responsive to the law, clinical studies may become larger and more expensive in order to be in compliance, with no guarantee that this is either the most efficient or effective way to advance the health interests of women or other groups. If this results in an inability to fund an adequate range of biomedical research, it is likely that the health interests of all people will suffer, and thus justice will not be served.

As part of the registry of clinical studies it is currently evaluating, NIH should establish a database cross-referenced by: (1) categories of disease and physiological or psychological factors and (2) study population composition of ongoing and published studies. This database should be compiled in a way that ensures easy accessibility to the data included by subgroup classification. Reporting requirements for all studies should be comprehensive and uniform and at a minimum include: the research questions addressed and the gender, race, ethnicity, socioeconomic status, age and hormonal status (i.e., pregnancy, stage of menstrual cycle) of the study population.

**To facilitate the collection of data about inclusion and justice from non-federally supported research, NIH should encourage journal publishers to require presentation of data on demographic characteristics.** Currently, there is no national norm that compels pharmaceutical manufacturers and other investigators to submit their data to a registry or other data repository.

**NIH should assist investigators in the effort to detect gender differences by: (1) identifying, developing, and disseminating alternative methods for detecting or formulating hypotheses about gender differences and (2) providing guidance for the use of these methods by investigators, IRGs, and TEGs.** The new legislative mandate makes it especially critical that both investigators and review committees clearly understand the interrelationship of sample sizes and the power to draw statistically significant inferences about differences between subgroups. A proactive strategy of development and dissemination would help investigators in complying with regulations. It would also help to prevent the introduction into the literature of analyses based on insufficient data—analyses that could ultimately do a disservice to subgroups by fostering seemingly valid but erroneous conclusions.

# Appendixes

# A

# Reports on Women's Participation in Clinical Studies, 1977-1993

**Sex as Reported in a Recent Sample of Psychological Research**
P. Reardon and S. Prescott (1977) *Psychology of Women Quarterly* 2(2):157-160.

> The authors reviewed all of the articles that appeared in the *Journal of Personality and Social Psychology*, volume 30, 1974, for sex of subjects, type of conclusions drawn, and whether sex was mentioned in the abstract, introduction, or methods section. These results were compared with those from a similar study done in 1972 in order to determine whether changes had occurred during the two-year period in scientific sampling and reporting procedures. The authors found that the percentage of all-male studies had dropped 15 percent while all-female studies had risen 22 percent. In addition, there was an increase in the number of both-sex studies that included some analysis of gender differences.

**Why Researchers Don't Study Women: The Responses of 62 Researchers**
S. Prescott (1978) *Sex Roles* 4(6):899-905.

> The author interviewed 62 researchers who had authored 64 single-sex studies appearing in the *Journal of Personality and Social Psychology* in 1970 and 1971 about their reasons for limiting their study population to males or females only. Replies were analyzed for thematic content and formed three major types: "scientific" (e.g., "desire to reduce the

variation in subjects' responses": 56 percent), "practical" (e.g., "limited money and resources for dealing with an increased sample size": 28 percent), and "extra-scientific" (e.g., "lack of interest in questions related to sex differences": 15 percent). The author concludes that there has been an imbalance in psychology which has led to the study of men rather than women or both sexes, and offers suggestions for counteracting gender-biased trends in psychological research and reporting.

## Underrepresentation of Women in New Drug Trials
E. L. Kinney, J. Trautmann, J. A. Gold, E. S. Vesell, and R. Zelis (1981) *Annals of Internal Medicine* 95(4):495-499.

This article presents findings of a survey of age and gender distribution of subjects participating in 50 clinical trials reported in 1979. The data indicate that young women served less frequently than young men as subjects in premarketing clinical drug trials. Moral, legal, and medical implications of this "underrepresentation" of women are considered; remedies to increase participation of young, nonpregnant women in clinical trials are discussed.

## National Institutes of Health: Problems in Implementing Policy on Women in Study Populations
General Accounting Office, Statement of M. V. Nadel (18 June 1990)

In this report, the General Accounting Office (GAO) reported that NIH had not successfully implemented its 1986 policy regarding the inclusion of women in clinical studies. As part of a necessarily informal study (because of the absence of organized data), the GAO reviewed 50 recent NIH grant applications, most of which proposed studies of conditions that affect both men and women. The GAO found that approximately 20 percent of the proposals provided no information on the sex of the study population. Over one-third of the proposals indicated that both men and women would be included, but did not specify in what proportions. In addition, a number of proposals for studies involving only male subjects provided no rationale for the single-sex design.

## Some Drug Trials Show Gender Bias
C. Hooper (1990) *Journal of NIH Research* 2:47-48.

This brief article describes data presented by researcher Dinah Reitman at the 1989 annual meeting of the American Public Health Association. Reitman compared the percentage of women enrolled in five categories of randomized control trials with the percentage of women affected by the corresponding medical conditions. In trials for AIDS drugs, Reitman found that the percentages were fairly close. In trials of nicotine gum for smoking cessation, she found that women were slightly "overrepresented." In three other therapeutic areas, however, Reitman found that women were "underrepresented" in clinical studies: antiplatelet drugs for preventing stroke, drugs for mild hypertension, and drugs for myocardial infarction.

## Women's Health Issues
National Heart, Lung, and Blood Institute (1990)

This publication outlines the past, present, and future of the NHLBI's acquisition and use of new knowledge about how cardiovascular disease affects women. It describes the Institute's efforts to recruit women as investigators in its research and training programs and as subjects in its clinical trials. Of the 18 NHLBI-initiated epidemiologic studies and primary prevention clinical trials active in 1990:

- 2 included exclusively women;
- 3 included between 30 and 45 percent women;
- 10 included between 50 and 58 percent women;
- 3 included exclusively men.

## Is There Still Too Much Extrapolation from Data on Middle-Aged White Men?
P. Cotton (1990) *Journal of the American Medical Association* 263(8):1049-1050.

The author describes how "efforts to streamline studies by using the most homogeneous population possible have filled medical libraries with data on middle-aged white men." He cites as examples the Multiple Risk-Factor Intervention Trial in 15,000 men, the Physician's Health Study (of aspirin's prophylactic effect in cardiovascular disease) of 22,071 men, and "all the large trials of cholesterol-lowering drugs," which include only men. Important gaps remain, the author notes, despite mounting documentation of important differences in drug responses and risk profiles among women, the elderly, and nonwhite persons.

## Most Major Companies Test Medicines in Women, Monitor Data for Gender Differences
L. E. Edwards (1991) In: *In Development: New Medicines for Women*, Pharmaceutical Manufacturers Association (December)

The author sent a survey to vice presidents of regulatory affairs at 46 pharmaceutical companies; 33 (including almost every major company) responded. All 33 companies reported that they collect data on gender of trial participants (94 percent always; 6 percent usually). Seventy-six percent of the companies reported that they deliberately recruit "representative" numbers of women for clinical trials.

## Sex, Trials, and Datatapes

R. S. Ungerleider and M. A. Friedman (1991) *Journal of the National Cancer Institute* 83(1): 16-17.

The authors examined the representation of women in federally funded clinical studies conducted by the National Cancer Institute's Clinical Trials Cooperative Group Program. In the repertoire of 444 treatment protocols active in January 1991, the only studies that specified gender were those for cancers that occur exclusively in one sex (with the exception of breast cancer protocols, which excluded men). Data from 1989 showed that 57% of all Phase II and Phase III study participants were female. The authors also noted that more women than men entered NCI clinical trials in 1989. During that year, 1.7 percent of all patients with newly diagnosed cancer entered Cooperative Group clinical trials; this total represents 2 percent of women and 1.5 percent of men with newly diagnosed cancer. The authors conclude that women are not "underrepresented" as subjects in federally funded studies conducted by NCI's Clinical Trials Cooperative Group Program.

## Assessing Future Research Needs: Mental and Addictive Disorders in Women

Summary of an Institute of Medicine Conference (October 1991)

Excerpt includes discussion of inclusion of women in ADAMHA-supported research. The internal ADAMHA working group on women's health reviewed 907 grants and found that women represented 53 percent of the population of subjects participating in these 907 studies.

## In Development: New Medicines for Women

Pharmaceutical Manufacturers Association (December 1991)

This 1991 survey found that 263 drugs were (at that time) being developed for use in women. The top three areas of drug development were cancer (58 medicines), gynecologic diseases (51 medicines), and cardiovascular/cerebrovascular disease (48 medicines). With 79 companies involved in these research projects, the PMA states that "virtually every major pharmaceutical company" is addressing the need to develop medicines that take into account the special medical needs of women. More than

50 percent of the research projects listed in this report were (at the time) in their final stages of development.

## Bridging the Gender Gap in Research
B. A. Levey (1991) *Clinical Pharmacology & Therapeutics* 50:641-646.

The author conducted a "spot comparison" of clinical trials reported in the January 1981 and 1991 issues of *Clinical Pharmacology & Therapeutics (CP&T)* and found a decline in the number of trials restricted to male subjects and a more than doubling of the number of trials that included both men and women. When the author extended the survey to clinical trials reported in all January issues of *CP&T* between 1981 and 1991, no consistent pattern (i.e., increase or decrease) emerged for trials that included both men and women. The author concluded that further investigation was required to conclude definitely that there had been a true progression toward an appropriate balance of men and women as research participants in trials published in *CP&T* in the past decade.

## Wanted: Single, White Male for Medical Research
R. Dresser (1992) *Hastings Center Report* (Jan/Feb):24-29.

The author claims that the failure to include women in research populations is "ubiquitous." She cites large-scale NIH-sponsored studies of heart attacks and aspirin, aging and health, caffeine and heart disease, and AIDS drugs, and even on obesity and breast and uterine cancer that have completely excluded women. The author also notes the "underrepresentation" of racial and ethnic minorities in clinical studies.

## Exclusion of Certain Groups from Clinical Research
E. Larson (In press) *Image: Journal of Nursing Scholarship*

This paper is a descriptive, retrospective review of research protocols approved by an IRB at a major tertiary care center during a two-year (1989, 1990) period. The review focuses on demographic characteristics of subjects and was conducted using exclusions specified in the written protocols. The author found in this review that women were not "underrepresented" in clinical drug trials or other types of research. She concluded that age, race, and socioeconomic status were more likely than gender to be associated with an unjustified exclusion from research protocols—the elderly, poor, and minority groups are excluded unjustifiably from research protocols.

**Sex Bias in Psychological Research: Progress or Complacency?**
L. Gannon, T. Luchetta, K. Rhodes, L. Pardie, and D. Segrist (1992) *American Psychologist* (March):389-396.

A total of 4,952 articles published in sample years between 1970 and 1990 in the areas of developmental, clinical, physiological, and social psychology were reviewed for the purpose of assessing various indicators of sexism in human psychological research. Significant changes in sex of first author, sex of participants, sexist language, and inappropriate generalization indicated to the authors that sexism has diminished in the past two decades. Despite these improvements, however, the authors conclude that the data revealed continued evidence of discriminatory practices.

**The Exclusion of the Elderly and Women from Clinical Trials in Acute Myocardial Infarction**
J. H. Gurwitz, N. F. Col, and J. Avorn (1992) *Journal of the American Medical Association* 268(11):1417-1422.

The authors conducted a systematic search of the English-language literature from January 1960 through September 1991 to identify all relevant studies of specific pharmacotherapies employed in the treatment of acute myocardial infarction. They searched MEDLINE, major cardiology textbooks, meta-analyses, reviews, editorials, and the bibliographies of all identified articles. They conclude that age-based exclusions are frequently used in clinical trials of medications used in the treatment of acute myocardial infarction and that such exclusions limit the ability to generalize study findings to the patient population that experiences the most morbidity and mortality from acute myocardial infarction: persons over age 75 (60 percent of deaths from acute myocardial infarction occur in persons over this age). And, since women outlive men by an average of 7.5 years, they are disproportionately represented in the elderly population. Furthermore, the authors found that studies with age-based exclusions had a smaller percentage of women compared with those without such exclusions.

**In Development: AIDS Medicines, Drugs, and Vaccines**
Pharmaceutical Manufacturers Association (October 1992)

With the dramatic increase in cases of AIDS in women, as well as its continued incidence in children, this PMA survey has identified clinical trials that focus on meeting the specific requirements of women and children with AIDS. The survey results show that there are 50 medicines in development that include women in the human clinical trials and 13 medicines that include children. The survey also indicates whether products will be specially labeled for use by women and/or children.

## Women's Health: FDA Needs to Ensure More Study of Gender Differences in Prescription Drug Testing
General Accounting Office (19 October 1992)

This publication reports the results of a GAO survey of pharmaceutical industry practices regarding inclusion of women in clinical trials. It concludes that:

- A quarter of drug manufacturers in the survey reported that they do not deliberately recruit "representative" numbers of women as participants in drug trials.
- Women were included in clinical trials for all drugs in the survey but were generally "underrepresented" in those trials.
- There were not enough women involved in the surveyed trials to detect gender related differences in response.
- Even when enough women are included in drug testing, often trial data are not analyzed to determine if women's responses to a drug differed from those of men.

## Women in AIDS and Orphan Drug Trials
Pharmaceutical Manufacturers Association (October 1992)

Another short newsbrief relating FDA testimony at the October 5th FDLI conference. Marlene Haffner, director of FDA's Office of Orphan Products Development noted that 26 products designated as orphans are in development for diseases that exclusively or predominantly affect women. And because orphan drugs are governed by the same guidelines and regulations as other drugs, Haffner noted, "enrollment of women is pretty much along the lines of the prevalence of the disease in women." Dianne Murphy of the FDA's Center for Drug Evaluation & Research noted that more women are being actively recruited into HIV trials. Women are in some Phase I trials, she added, and some studies even include pregnant women.

## Sexism in a Leading Medical Journal—A Quantitative Measure
K. Williams and E. F. Manace Borins (1993) *Journal of the American Women's Medical Association* 48(5):160-162.

The authors examined 160 randomly selected articles from the 1989 *New England Journal of Medicine*. Each article was coded using a differentiated analysis of gender bias. Sixteen components of the research process were examined. Significant (present in greater than 60 percent of the articles) gender bias was found in 12 of the 16 components. The authors conclude that medical research in 1989 was still seriously gender-biased, and therefore scientifically flawed.

## Understanding the Second Epidemic: The Status of Research on Women and AIDS in the United States
H. Pham, P. Freeman, and N. Kohn (1992) Center for Women Policy Studies, Washington, D.C.

A report from the Center for Women Policy Studies that makes recommendations for woman-focused HIV/AIDS research. The report states that women, intravenous drug users, people of color, and people of low income have been "grossly underrepresented" among study subjects in ACTG clinical trials. It cites two barriers to women's participation in clinical trials: (1) many HIV-positive women had not developed a clinical diagnosis of CDC-defined AIDS and (2) federal regulations placing special emphasis on the avoidance of potential risks to fetuses.

## Memo to Human Subjects Committee re: Frequency of Exclusion of Fertile Women from Drug Studies
R. A. Charo (23 March 1992) Unpublished memo.
See also: **Restrictions on the Participation of Women in Drug Studies: A Retrospective Analysis,** R. A. Charo (1990), unpublished paper.

Based on an evaluation of all drug study protocols submitted for review to the Human Subjects Committee at the University of Wisconsin in 1989 and 1990, this memo provides data on the frequency of exclusion of women of reproductive age from these protocols. One hundred and sixty-nine new drug studies were reviewed (this number excluded Phase I studies, studies of male-only or postmenopause-only disorders, and studies of diseases in infants). Twenty-eight of the 169 studies (16.5 percent/1 in 6) excluded fertile women. Twenty-two of these 28 studies were sponsored by drug companies. The author also analyzed the data after separating out protocols involving cancer agents and other known fetotoxic drugs.

## Gender Bias in Medical Research
M. Eichler, A. L. Reisman, and E. Borins (1992) *Women and Therapy—A Feminist Quarterly* 12(4):61-71.

The authors apply a system of identifying gender bias in research to selected 1988 issues of medical journals representing various subspecialties of medical research: the *New England Journal of Medicine*, the *Canadian Journal of Surgery*, the *American Journal of Trauma*, and the

*American Journal of Psychiatry*. The authors state that no particular method was used in selecting the journal issues; their intent was not to compare gender bias in different subspecialties or publication outlets, but to provide recent examples of gender bias in medical research. They conclude that gender bias in medical research is pervasive.

## Citizen's Petition to the Food and Drug Administration: Statement of Grounds
NOW Legal Defense and Education Fund (February 1993)

This statement describes the level of participation of women in AIDS Clinical Trial Group (ACTG) clinical trials. It states that although the percentage of female enrollment in these trials increased from 6.5 percent to 7.8 percent from 1990 to 1992, the numbers of women enrolled are inadequate to provide sound, meaningful data on the effects of a given drug on women. It cites the even greater exclusion of pregnant women from clinical trials: In a review of 74 AIDS clinical trials open for enrollment in New York and New Jersey in October 1990, 57 (80 percent) excluded pregnant women.

## Women's Access to Government-Sponsored AIDS/HIV Clinical Trials: Status Report, Critique, and Recommendations
I. L. Long (March 1993) Prepared for the NIH/ORWH Public Hearing on the Recruitment and Retention of Women in Clinical Trials

The author argues that women with AIDS/HIV disease have been explicitly or implicitly excluded from most clinical trials, whether sponsored by the government or by pharmaceutical manufacturers. She provides data indicating that women are not represented in ACTU (AIDS Clinical Unit) trials proportionately with their reported incidence of AIDS. She also argues that people of color are "underrepresented" in most trials.

## Determinants of Accrual of Women to a Large, Multicenter HIV/AIDS Clinical Trials Program in the United States
D. J. Cotton, W. He, J. Feinberg, and D. M. Finkelstein (1993) *Journal of Acquired Immune Deficiency* 6:1322-1328.

The authors describe their efforts to determine factors influencing enrollment of women in a large, multicenter clinical trials program in the United States, including attributes of participants, sites, and the trials themselves. They found that women accounted for 6.7 percent of the 11,909 AIDS Clinical Trials Group (ACTG) participants from 1987 through 1990. Women entering ACTG trials were significantly more likely to be white and less likely to have ever used intravenous drugs than U.S. women reported with AIDS. The authors conclude that the low enrollment of women in general in these trials was influenced by demographic and geographic factors rather than attributes of specific trials. They note that an apparent positive influence of female research unit leadership on increasing enrollment of women merits further study.

**Memo to Co-chairs of the NAS/IOM Committee on Legal and Ethical Issues Relating to the Inclusion of Women in Clinical Studies re: Johns Hopkins University IRB Counts**
C. L. Meinert (14 April 1993)

Dr. Meinert reports on his survey of proposals approved by IRBs at the Johns Hopkins University. Dr. Meinert's survey included all active proposals, proposals pending further action by the IRB, and proposals reviewed and approved and completed or terminated within the last two years. Of a total of 2,801 proposals, 181 involved males only (6.5 percent), 265 involved females only (9.5 percent), and 2,355 (84 percent) involved both males and females.

**Memo to Co-chairs of the NAS/IOM Committee on the Legal and Ethical Issues Relating to the Inclusion of Women in Clinical Studies re: NIH Inventory of Clinical Trials**
C. L. Meinert (5 May 1993)

Of 293 trials listed in the 1979 NIH inventory of clinical trials, all but 25 involved both males and females. Of the 25 involving only males or females, 13 involved females and 12 involved males. All 12 of the exclusively female trials involved uniquely or primarily female conditions, whereas only 4 of the 12 exclusively male trials involved uniquely or primarily male conditions. [Note: see Dickersin and Min (1993) NIH clinical trials and publication bias. *Online Journal of Current Clinical Trials* doc. 50 (28 April), in which the authors examined the same data and came to similar conclusions.]

**Memo to Co-chairs of the NAS/IOM Committee on the Legal and Ethical Issues Relating to the Inclusion of Women in Clinical Studies re: Clinical Trials in *Controlled Clinical Trials***
C. L. Meinert (5 May 1993)

Meinert describes the findings of his survey of the reported gender and ethnic mix of trials published in a journal, *Controlled Clinical Trials,* from its inception to the present. Of a total of 38 papers describing actual clinical trials, only 28 provided explicit statements regarding gender inclusion criteria, and among those 28, only 21 provided exact counts of males and females. The 21 trials involved a total sample size of 78,840, of whom 72,951 were males and 5,890 were females. The results provide some evidence for a predilection for male-based trials, at least among those authors electing to publish in this journal (or perhaps among the journal's editors). There was very little information about the ethnic mix of the trial populations.

**Letter to Curtis Meinert Regarding Gender Representation in NEI Clinical Trials**
National Eye Institute; National Institutes of Health (20 May 1993)

The letter states that significant numbers of women are included in a variety of NEI-supported trials. In almost all NEI trials, women comprise at least 40 percent of the participants. Women represent 77 percent of the subject population in trials for treatments of optical neuritis, a condition known to be more prevalent in women than in men.

**Memo to Co-chairs of the NAS/IOM Committee on Legal and Ethical Issues Relating to the Inclusion of Women in Clinical Studies re: On Gender Coverage at Johns Hopkins University**
C. L. Meinert (21 May 1993)

This memo describes an analysis of gender-specific studies at Johns Hopkins University that were identified in a previous memo (14 April). Gender-specific studies were classified as to whether or not the focus on one gender has a biological or disease basis, as determined by the title of the project. A higher percentage of male-only studies were found to be arbitrarily male-only, as opposed to female-only studies that were arbitrarily female-only (75.2 percent and 21.2 percent, respectively). Also found was a greater propensity to study females than males overall (3:1), as well as reproductive or sex-specific diseases (47:1 and 6:1, respectively).

**Letter to Curtis Meinert Regarding Gender Representation in Clinical Trials Performed by the National Heart, Lung, and Blood Institute**
National Heart, Lung, and Blood Institute (26 May 1993)

This memo describes data that Dr. Meinert received from the director of the National Heart, Lung, and Blood Institute in response to his request for information about clinical trials under way at the Institute. The figures are as of May 1993. They include a total of 49 trials, one of which is being done in males only and eight of which are being done in females only. The gender mix in the remaining trials ranges from a low of about 10 percent female to about 75 percent female.

**Women's Representation as Subjects in Clinical Studies: A Pilot Study of Research Published in *JAMA* in 1990 and 1992** (in Volume 2 of this report)

C.E. Bird (May 1993) Paper prepared for the IOM Committee on the Legal and Ethical Issues Relating to the Inclusion of Women in Clinical Studies

In this study, all original articles reporting results of clinical studies in two recent years (1990 and 1992) of the *Journal of the American Medical Association* (*JAMA*) were examined (see commissioned paper by Bird for full details). Articles were classified by the percent of women included as subjects (grouped into five categories: 0 percent, 1 percent<x<33 percent, 34 percent<x<66 percent, 67 percent<x<99 percent, 100 percent), by major disease/treatment category, and by major design methodology. Two definitions of gender underrepresentation were used: a "strict" definition: 0 percent (either gender) and a "lenient" definition: one-third or fewer (either gender). There were 243 articles that met the definition of a clinical study and had enough information to classify gender of their subjects. Of these, 207 related to gender-neutral diseases (disease can occur in both genders). The results reported here pertain to these 207 articles studying gender-neutral diseases. (Note: "gender-neutral" disease as used in this study does not imply that the incidence of disease is equal in both genders, but merely that it is reasonably common in both genders. Breast cancer, for example, is not considered to be gender-neutral because it occurs very rarely among men.)

Among clinical studies studying gender-neutral diseases, 49 percent had samples with women representing between one-third and two-thirds of their subjects. Among the remaining 51 percent, there was some fairly strong evidence to suggest that women were more likely to be underrepresented as research subjects compared with underrepresentation of men. Specifically, 17 percent of the studies had no women compared with 6 percent with no men (ratio of 4.3); 38 percent had one-third or fewer women subjects compared with 14 percent with one-third or fewer men (ratio of 2.7).

There were three types of methodological designs with at least 40 articles concerning gender-neutral diseases: cross-sectional (45), longitudinal (100), and RCTs (40). For all three types of designs, about 50 percent had samples with women representing between one-third and two-thirds of their subjects. For simplicity's sake, the remaining articles are presented as the ratio of those which underrepresent women to those which underrepresent men. Using the strict definition of underrepresentation, this ratio was 0.8 for cross-sectional studies, 3.6 for longitudinal studies, and 5.0 for RCTs. Using the lenient definition, this ratio was 2.5 for cross-sectional, 2.8 for longitudinal, and 3.4 for RCT studies. Thus, there was some evidence to suggest that there are some systematic differences among design methodologies if the strict definition is used (with RCTs being most likely to exclude women in comparison to excluding men), a tendency that was reduced when the lenient definition was used.

One reason for underrepresentation of women in gender-neutral diseases may be that the disease is less common among women than men. Using the strict definition of underrepresentation, the 46 single-gender studies examining gender-neutral diseases were categorized by the primary basis for excluding one gender: prevalence (for example, the disease occurs disproportionately in one gender or the particular vector or risk factor of interest was gender-specific), convenience (for example, the population was veterans or prisoners, data gathering was easier in one sex, secondary analysis of data from sex-specific study), or no discernible rationale.

Several findings emerged. First, overall, the choice of single-gender populations could be rationalized by either the prevalence of the disease or sampling convenience in most instances (over 85 percent). The remaining 15 percent of studies had no apparent rationale, either offered by the authors or inferred on the basis of the disease or site of study. This percentage remained about the same for both subsets of male-only and female-only studies as well. Female-only and male-only studies, however, appeared to differ systematically by whether the basis of the choice was disease prevalence (75 percent of female-only studies compared with 41 percent of male-only studies) or convenience (8 percent of female-only studies compared with 47 percent of male-only studies). Partial explanations for this imbalance were that 53 percent of all studies for which convenience was the primary basis examined the (almost exclusively male) veteran population and another 24 percent of these studies consisted of secondary analyses of single-gender studies, which tended to be all-male.

These findings suggest that one important reason for a tendency for male-only studies to predominate is the differential opportunity for men to be in positions where clinical studies are likely to be funded and carried out (for example, receiving treatment in a Veterans Administration Medical Center or as a member of the armed services or as a prisoner) which in turn can create further imbalance as researchers seek to take advantage of databases already collected. Perhaps one way to redress this source of gender imbalance in clinical studies is to fund studies in institutional settings where women predominate, e.g., nursing homes, hospital employees, or primary grade teachers.

This study suggests that, among those studies examining gender-neutral diseases, women were more likely than men to be underrepresented. The reasons why women tend to be underrepresented—such as incidence of the disease by gender or convenience of samples by site, such as the Veteran Administration Medical Center population or men's prisons—may help explain the scientific rationale on a study-by-study basis. Nonetheless, viewed as a whole, there is evidence to suggest that the end-result of these individual decisions is to have fewer women in clinical studies of diseases common in both genders.

### Letter to Anna Mastroianni from Iris J. Schneider Regarding the Inclusion of Females and Males in Clinical Trials Supported by the National Cancer Institute
National Cancer Institute (23 June 1993)

This memo provides subject counts for NCI clinical trials in fiscal year 1992. Of 22,483 participants in treatment trials, 12,490 were females and 9,993 were males. Of 9,553 participants in prevention trials, 4,727 were females and 4,826 were males. No information is provided regarding the conditions studied.

### Women in Clinical Trials: HIV-Infected Women
D. Murphy (1993) *Food and Drug Law Journal* 48(2): 175-179.

This article summarizes a presentation given by the author at the Food and Drug Law Institute's seminar, "Women in Clinical Trials of FDA-Regulated Products: Who Participates and Who Decides?" on October 5, 1992, in Washington, D.C. She notes that in 1991, 13 percent of reported AIDS cases occurred in females. As of August, 1992, females made up 13.2 percent of the total ACTG trial population. Of the adults in trials, women made up 10.7 percent. She describes the improvement in recruitment of women over time: where women made up 6.8 percent of the population in the first 20 ACTG protocols, but they made up 15.7 percent of the population in the last 20 ACTG trials, with significant enrollment numbers.

### Update on Clinical Trials and Pharmaceutical Regimens for Women with HIV Infection
J. A. Korvick and I. Long (1993) In *Until the Cure: Caregiving for Women with HIV*, A. Kurth, ed.

An analysis from the National Institute of Allergy and Infectious Diseases (NIAID) Division of AIDS. The authors report that the number of females in ACTG clinical trials increased from 2 percent in 1986 to over 18 percent in 1992.

## Guideline for the Study and Evaluation of Gender Differences in the Clinical Evaluation of Drugs; Notice

Food and Drug Administration (1993) *Federal Register* 58 (139):39412 (22 July 1993)

In this notice of proposed policy revision, the FDA noted that the effect of the 1977 guideline that excluded women of childbearing potential from participation in early studies of drugs has been that women generally have not been included in Phase I nontherapeutic studies or in the earliest controlled effectiveness (Phase II) studies except for studies of life-threatening illnesses. The notice includes accounts of FDA surveys of new drug applications (NDAs) undertaken in 1983 and 1989. These are summarized below:

*Food and Drug Administration Survey of New Drug Applications (NDAs), 1983*

Carried out primarily to assess the inclusion of elderly persons in new drug applications (NDAs), this survey examined the age and gender of patient populations included in 11 pending NDAs. The NDAs were chosen because they were readily available and did not need to be retrieved from storage. The survey showed that nonsteroidal anti-inflammatory drugs were studied predominantly in women (because arthritis is more common in women), that this predominance was slightly less in the case of a pain medication, and that a hypnotic drug and two antibiotics were studied in equal proportions of men and women. The patient populations in the NDAs for two drugs to treat heart disease were about two-thirds male. About two-thirds of the patients in these studies were less than 60 years of age, an age group in which heart disease is more prevalent in men than women. In patients over 70, the gender distribution was about equal. Studies of a drug to treat duodenal ulcer, a predominantly male condition, included about 75 percent males. The two anti-cancer drugs in the survey were studied principally for exclusively male conditions, prostate cancer and testis cancer.

*Food and Drug Administration Survey of NDAs, 1988*

In an effort to examine selection bias, the FDA surveyed all drugs approved in 1988 (with the exception of 4 orphan drugs, 3 contrast agents for single dose uses, and a topical product for which gender distribution was not available). Study populations for an anti-inflammatory drug and a drug for prevention of vascular spasm after subarachnoid hemorrhage (both female-predominant conditions) were primarily female. Studies of two cardiovascular drugs included 59 and 67 percent men, reflecting the predominance of angina, "and perhaps hypertension," in men under age 60 (two-thirds of patients were under age 60). An intravenous antibiotic was studied mainly in elderly patients; for unknown reasons, about two-thirds of the patients studied were male. One topical was also studied somewhat more in males for unknown reasons.

## Underrepresentation of Women in Clinical Drug Trials
D. L. Schmucker and E. S. Vesell (1993) *Clinical Pharmacology & Therapeutics* 54:11-15.

The authors performed a quantitative survey of gender distribution in test populations of trials reported in all issues of *Clinical Pharmacology and Therapeutics* (*CP&T*) during the periods from 1969 to 1971, 1979 to 1981, and 1989 to 1991, and the *British Journal of Clinical Pharmacology* (*BJCP*) during the periods from 1979 to 1981 and 1989 to 1991—an interval encompassing 22 years and including 1,947 articles. Not included in the survey were trials on contraceptives or drugs designed for gender-specific diseases or conditions, case histories, and single-subject trials. The authors found that the percentage of trials reported in *CP&T* that included men only increased from 27 percent to 38 percent from 1969-1971 to 1989-1991. A similar comparison in the *BJCP* from 1979-1981 to 1989-1991 yielded a 5 percent increase. In both journals during these same periods, the percentage of women-only trials declined. In neither journal was there a statistically significant increase in the percentage of trials that included both men and women. During these same periods, the number of trials that did not declare subject gender decreased by 57 percent in *CP&T* and 23 percent in *BJCP*.

To estimate the frequency of gender-related differences in drug effects, the authors surveyed all clinical trials published in *CP&T* during 1991 that included both men and women for documented gender differences in drug responses. There were 68 such trials, and none claimed differences in drug response that were attributable to gender. The majority of trials (>60 percent) failed to mention whether or not the data were analyzed for gender differences.

The authors also examined for gender-related differences in efficacy or toxicity all drugs approved by the FDA in 1981 and 1991 and that were listed in the 1992 *Physicians Desk Reference* (*PDR*). Data cited under the headings of Clinical Pharmacology, Contraindications, Precautions, and Adverse Reactions were reviewed for recommendations for restricted use of the drug in nonpregnant women and pregnant women. The survey revealed reservations concerning use during pregnancy, but not in nonpregnant women, for nearly all drugs approved in 1981 and 1991. The authors note that the values are difficult to interpret, however, because absence of any contraindications for drug use in nonpregnant women may reflect (1) no evidence of gender differences, (2) exclusion of women from test populations, or (3) failure to analyze clinical trial data for gender differences. The authors conclude that despite efforts to rectify the underrepresentation of women as participants in clinical trials, this practice has continued during the past decade.

## The Right to Participate in Research Studies
M. L. Elks (1993) *Journal of Laboratory and Clinical Medicine* 122:130-136.

The author reviewed three journals to determine the proportion of women in clinical (nongonadal) studies. In volume 51 of *Clinical Pharmacology & Therapeutics* (January through June 1992, chosen because of publication of clinical studies of new drugs), 49 studies were reported; 14 (29 percent) included no women and 2 (4 percent) included no men; none of these articles noted this exclusionary status in the titles. The remaining 26 studies had an average of 59 percent male participants. In volume 263 of the *American Journal of Physiology: Endocrinology and Metabolism* (July through November 1992, chosen because of studies of metabolism/physiology), 32 studies were reported, with 10 (31 percent) including only men (one so stating in the title), 1 (3 percent) including only women, and 4 (12.5 percent) giving no statement of the gender of participants. The 16 remaining studies had an average of 57 percent male participants. In volume 19 of *Hypertension* (January through June 1992, chosen because hypertension is more common in women than in men), 20 studies were reported; 8 (40 percent) included no women (one title so stated) and 3 were large epidemiologic studies with equal representation. The 9 remaining studies had an average of 64 percent male participants. In the 38 rat studies in this journal, 7 did not state the sex of the rats, 26 (68 percent) used males only, 1 (3 percent) used females only, and 4 (11 percent) included both. None of the titles indicated the gender of the animals studied. The author concludes that frequent systematic exclusion of females has occurred both in human and animal studies. The author also notes that even in most of the both-sex studies, notably more men than women have been included than would be likely by chance.

**Inclusion of Women and Minorities in Occupational Cancer Epidemiological Research**
Zahm, S.H., Pottern, L.M., Lewis, D.R., Ward, M.H., and White, D.W. (In press). Submitted to *Journal of Occupational Medicine.*

Of a total of 1,233 studies, 562 (46 percent) included only white men, while the remaining 671 studies (54 percent) included subjects from other race-gender groups. Of these, 35 percent included white women, but only 14 percent presented any analyses of the white women specifically. The proportions with analyses of non-white women (any: 2 percent; detailed: 1 percent) or non-white men (any: 7 percent; detailed: 3 percent) were also small. Studies with detailed analyses of women and minorities tended to use weaker methodologies (i.e., proportionate mortality or cross-sectional design) than the studies of white men and were less able to provide convincing data on the occupational cancer risks of women and minorities.

# B

# NIH Revitalization Act of 1993
# Public Law 103-43

# Subtitle B—Clinical Research Equity Regarding Women and Minorities

## PART I—WOMEN AND MINORITIES AS SUBJECTS IN CLINICAL RESEARCH

**SEC. 131. REQUIREMENT OF INCLUSION IN RESEARCH.**

Part G of title IV of the Public Health Service Act, as amended by section 101 of this Act, is amended by inserting after section 492A the following section:

"INCLUSION OF WOMEN AND MINORITIES IN CLINICAL RESEARCH

"SEC. 492B. (a) REQUIREMENT OF INCLUSION.—

"(1) IN GENERAL.—In conducting or supporting clinical research for purposes of this title, the Director of NIH shall, subject to subsection (b), ensure that—

"(A) women are included as subjects in each project of such research; and

"(B) members of minority groups are included as subjects in such research.

"(2) OUTREACH REGARDING PARTICIPATION AS SUBJECTS.—The Director of NIH, in consultation with the Director of the Office of Research on Women's Health and the Director of the Office of Research on Minority Health, shall conduct or support outreach programs for the recruitment of women and members of minority groups as subjects in projects of clinical research.

"(b) INAPPLICABILITY OF REQUIREMENT.—The requirement established in subsection (a) regarding women and members of minority groups shall not apply to a project of clinical research if the inclusion, as subjects in the project, of women and members of minority groups, respectively—

"(1) is inappropriate with respect to the health of the subjects;

"(2) is inappropriate with respect to the purpose of the research; or

"(3) is inappropriate under such other circumstances as the Director of NIH may designate.

"(c) DESIGN OF CLINICAL TRIALS.—In the case of any clinical trial in which women or members of minority groups will under subsection (a) be included as subjects, the Director of NIH shall ensure that the trial is designed and carried out in a manner sufficient to provide for a valid analysis of whether the variables being studied in the trial affect women or members of minority groups, as the case may be, differently than other subjects in the trial.

"(d) GUIDELINES.—

"(1) IN GENERAL.—Subject to paragraph (2), the Director of NIH, in consultation with the Director of the Office of Research on Women's Health and the Director of the Office of Research on Minority Health, shall establish guidelines regarding the requirements of this section. The guidelines shall include guidelines regarding—

"(A) the circumstances under which the inclusion of women and minorities as subjects in projects of clinical research is inappropriate for purposes of subsection (b);

"(B) the manner in which clinical trials are required to be designed and carried out for purposes of subsection (c); and

"(C) the operation of outreach programs under subsection (a).

"(2) CERTAIN PROVISIONS.—With respect to the circumstances under which the inclusion of women or members of minority groups (as the case may be) as subjects in a project of clinical research is inappropriate for purposes of subsection (b), the following applies to guidelines under paragraph (1):

"(A)(i) In the case of a clinical trial, the guidelines shall provide that the costs of such inclusion in the trial is not a permissible consideration in determining whether such inclusion is inappropriate.

"(ii) In the case of other projects of clinical research, the guidelines shall provide that the costs of such inclusion in the project is not a permissible consideration in determining whether such inclusion is inappropriate unless the data regarding women or members of minority groups, respectively, that would be obtained in such project (in the event that such inclusion were required) have been or are being obtained through other means that provide data of comparable quality.

"(B) In the case of a clinical trial, the guidelines may provide that such inclusion in the trial is not required if there is substantial scientific data demonstrating that there is no significant difference between—

"(i) the effects that the variables to be studied in the trial have on women or members of minority groups, respectively; and

"(ii) the effects that the variables have on the individuals who would serve as subjects in the trial in the event that such inclusion were not required.

"(e) DATE CERTAIN FOR GUIDELINES; APPLICABILITY.—

"(1) DATE CERTAIN.—The guidelines required in subsection (d) shall be established and published in the Federal Register not later than 180 days after the date of the enactment of the National Institutes of Health Revitalization Act of 1993.

"(2) APPLICABILITY.—For fiscal year 1995 and subsequent fiscal years, the Director of NIH may not approve any proposal of clinical research to be conducted or supported by any agency of the National Institutes of Health unless the proposal specifies the manner in which the research will comply with this section.

"(f) REPORTS BY ADVISORY COUNCILS.—The advisory council of each national research institute shall prepare biennial reports describing the manner in which the institute has complied with this section. Each such report shall be submitted to the Director of the institute involved for inclusion in the biennial report under section 403.

"(g) DEFINITIONS.—For purposes of this section:

"(1) The term 'project of clinical research' includes a clinical trial.

"(2) The term 'minority group' includes subpopulations of minority groups. The Director of NIH shall, through the guidelines established under subsection (d), define the terms 'minority group' and 'subpopulation' for purposes of the preceding sentence.".

### SEC. 132. PEER REVIEW.

Section 492 of the Public Health Service Act (42 U.S.C. 289a) is amended by adding at the end the following subsection:

"(c)(1) In technical and scientific peer review under this section of proposals for clinical research, the consideration of any such proposal (including the initial consideration) shall, except as provided in paragraph (2), include an evaluation of the technical and scientific merit of the proposal regarding compliance with section 492B.

"(2) Paragraph (1) shall not apply to any proposal for clinical research that, pursuant to subsection (b) of section 492B, is not subject to the requirement of subsection (a) of such section regarding the inclusion of women and members of minority groups as subjects in clinical research.".

### SEC. 133. INAPPLICABILITY TO CURRENT PROJECTS.

Section 492B of the Public Health Service Act, as added by section 131 of this Act, shall not apply with respect to projects of clinical research for which initial funding was provided prior to the date of the enactment of this Act. With respect to the inclusion of women and minorities as subjects in clinical research conducted or supported by the National Institutes of Health, any policies of the Secretary of Health and Human Services regarding such inclusion that are in effect on the day before the date of the enactment of this Act shall continue to apply to the projects referred to in the preceding sentence.

# C

# DES Case Study

## HISTORY OF DEVELOPMENT AND TESTING OF DES

Diethylstilbestrol (DES) is a synthetic estrogen. It was first produced in London in 1938 and was prescribed from 1945 to 1971 to prevent spontaneous abortions (NIH, 1992). The earliest studies of DES in pregnant women in the United States were conducted at Harvard University in the late 1940s. Although the studies were criticized because they were conducted without the use of controls, the physicians directing the studies concluded that DES was effective against a variety of pregnancy complications and resulted in a healthier maternal environment (Weitzner and Hirsch, 1981). In 1947 the FDA approved new drug applications (NDAs) to market DES for the purpose of preventing miscarriages (Mascaro, 1991).

In the 1950s, however, controlled studies of DES in pregnant women yielded different results. At Tulane University, researchers found that more of the DES-treated women had miscarriages and premature births, while the controls had bigger, healthier babies. At the University of Chicago, every pregnant woman at the University's Lying-In Hospital became part of a clinical trial: one-half were randomized to receive DES and the other half received placebos. None of the women were told they were part of a study, nor were they told what drug they were taking. The study found that twice as many of the DES-treated mothers had miscarriages and small babies. Despite growing evidence that DES was ineffective, for the next 20 years the drug was administered to pregnant women to prevent miscarriage (Weitzner and Hirsch, 1981). In 1951 the FDA concluded that DES was safe for use during pregnancy and stopped requiring manufacturers to complete NDAs prior to marketing the drug as a preventive against miscarriage (Mascaro, 1991).

## DES-RELATED INJURIES

In 1971 an article in the *New England Journal of Medicine* reported that between 1966 and 1971 seven cases of clear-cell adenocarcinoma (CCA) had been found in teenage girls (Herbst et al., 1971). CCA is an extremely rare cancer, particularly in young women. The common element to these seven cases was that their mothers had taken DES during their pregnancies. In that same year, the FDA banned the use of DES as a miscarriage preventive; but by that time, an estimated 1.5 million babies had been exposed to DES. Thirty thousand were exposed in 1971 alone (Weitzner and Hirsch, 1981).

Research has found that DES interferes with the formation of normal genital tissue during fetal development. Many studies have found possible associations between DES exposure and abnormalities in daughters of women who took DES while pregnant. These studies, including one looking at DES daughters whose mothers were involved in the University of Chicago experiments, have found possible associations between DES exposure and vaginal and cervical dysplasia (a type of abnormal tissue that either reverts with time or progresses slowly to cancer); adenosis (glandular proliferation); cervical ridges and cervical erosion; uterine structural abnormalities, such as a T-shape of the endometrial cavity and/or an unusually small uterus; uterine hypoplasia (underdeveloped cells); infertility; menstrual irregularities; ectopic pregnancies; fetal death and premature birth; and breast and reproductive-tract cancers (Weitzner and Hirsch, 1981). The pathologic changes were more common in women exposed to high DES doses and those exposed early in gestation. It is estimated that there are almost two million "DES daughters" now of childbearing age (NIH, 1992).

Injury to male babies, or DES sons, has also been reported. No malignant tumors have been reported, but certain genital and semen abnormalities are more common in men exposed to DES in utero than in men not exposed to DES. These abnormalities include penile bleeding, testicular masses, epididymal cysts, hypoplastic testes, and cryptorchidism (undescended testicle) (NIH, 1992). One article reported that one in three DES sons is sterile (Weitzner and Hirsch, 1981). Other authors call for more studies to determine whether the observed abnormalities are correlated with an increased risk of infertility (NIH, 1992).

There have also been allegations of injury to third generations. Two legal actions were initiated on behalf of DES granddaughters who claim that their disabilities were caused by their premature birth, which resulted from damage to their mothers' reproductive organs from in utero DES exposure (see *Enright v. Eli Lilly & Co.* and *Sorrels v. Eli Lilly & Co.*). In addition, one DES son filed a legal action alleging that his teenage daughter's fatal case of clear-cell adenocarcinoma was caused by his exposure to DES in utero (Squires, 1991).

In addition to reproductive abnormalities, research in animals has shown that DES may induce certain autoimmune disorders. Two small studies done on humans have shown altered T-cell and natural killer cell function in women exposed in utero to DES, and data from one cohort of "DES daughters" shows an increase in reported incidence of autoimmune diseases. Whether DES exposure is associated with an increased risk of developing an autoimmune disorder is an active area of research (NIH, 1992). Concern over the effects of DES on persons exposed in utero continues to prompt further study. The National Cancer Institute (NCI) recently issued a request for applications (RFA) inviting cooperative agreement applications from investigators to assist NCI in studies of women with DES-associated clear-cell adenocarcinoma of the cervix or vagina (The Blue Sheet, 1993). Another RFA from NCI and the National Institute of Child Health and Human Development (NICHD) invites cooperative agreement applications to develop a national program to inform health professionals and the public on the adverse effects of DES (NIH, 1993). Initial awards for both RFAs were expected to be made in September 1993. In addition, an added $2.9 million in federal funds was recently allocated to fund further studies of health problems in DES sons, as well as in daughters and their mothers (Brody, 1993).

## LIABILITY

There have been numerous legal actions initiated by daughters whose mothers were exposed to DES during pregnancy; more than a thousand were pending nationwide as of February 1991 (Squires, 1991). Because over 300 companies manufactured DES according to the same formula and pharmacists often filled prescriptions at random, the chief barrier to recovery for most DES plaintiffs is identifying the manufacturer who supplied the drug that a particular mother ingested. Many of the successful cases have relied on theories of joint and several liability (Mascaro, 1991: 447).

There have been two reported cases coming out of the University of Chicago experiments in the 1950s. In *Mink v. University of Chicago*, three women filed an action against Eli Lilly, a pharmaceutical company manufacturing DES, and the University of Chicago to recover for their daughters' development of abnormal cervical cellular formations and for their daughters' increased risk of vaginal and cervical cancer. They also alleged that they themselves and their sons had suffered reproductive and other abnormalities and an increased cancer risk. In addition, the plaintiffs asked the court to allow them to represent the other women in the experiment who were given DES by certifying their case as a class action. The court declined to certify the case as a class action, but issued an opinion on whether the plaintiffs' claims of injury to themselves and their daughters had merit.

The plaintiffs claimed they were not told that they were part of an experiment, nor were they informed that they were taking DES. They also claimed that since the DES-cancer link was known by 1971, the manufacturer should be liable for making no effort to warn them until late 1975-1976. The plaintiffs maintained that the University had committed a battery by performing a medical experiment on them without their knowledge. They also asserted that the University had breached a duty to notify them that they had taken DES and that their children should be regularly examined. The plaintiffs claimed that Eli Lilly was strictly liable for the manufacture of a defective and unreasonably dangerous drug.

In a hearing on whether the case should be dismissed, the court held that Eli Lilly had a duty to notify the plaintiffs about the DES risks when the company became aware of them or should have become aware of them. Under Illinois tort law, however, in order for the plaintiffs to recover under theories of breach of duty to warn and in strict liability, they must allege physical injury to themselves. Because the plaintiffs in their complaint cited risk of injury or physical injuries to others (their children) under their claims of breach of duty to warn and strict liability, the court dismissed these complaints.

The court did not dismiss the battery allegations. The court held that performing nonemergency treatment without consent or knowledge is an unauthorized contact with another person, or a battery. The court stated that the resolution of the case would not turn on the issue of informed consent or whether there was incomplete disclosure of risks before consent was obtained; because there was a complete absence of consent, the issue to be resolved was whether the University had committed battery against these women (*Mink v. University of Chicago*).

The case was settled before trial, and the plaintiffs together received a monetary settlement of $225,000 from the University of Chicago for the battery claim. Although the court declined to certify the case as a class action, attorneys for the plaintiffs were able to get the University to agree to provide some services to the other women and their offspring as part of the settlement agreement. The University agreed to treat, free-of-charge, the daughters of any women involved in the 1950 experiments who develop DES-associated vaginal or cervical cancer. They also agreed to provide free annual or biannual medical exams for all offspring exposed to DES in utero during these experiments (Schultz, 1982).

In the second reported case of DES injury from the University of Chicago experiments, two DES daughters initiated legal action against the University of Chicago and Eli Lilly, alleging their injuries resulted from their mother's participation in the experiments while they were in utero. The plaintiffs also based their legal claims on theories of battery, strict liability, and breach of duty to warn/lack of informed consent. The case was settled out of court for an undisclosed amount (*Wetherill v. University of Chicago*).

## REFERENCES

The Blue Sheet. 1993. Follow-up of DES-associated clear cell adenocarcinoma. *The Blue Sheet* (14 April, Suppl.):6-7.

Brody, J.E. 1993. Adult years bring new afflictions for DES "babies." *New York Times,* February 10:B6, C12.

Herbst, A.L., Ulfelder, H., and Poskanzer, D.C. 1971. Adenocarcinoma of the vagina. Association of maternal stilbestrol therapy with tumor appearance in young women. *New England Journal of Medicine* 284(15):878-881.

Keeton, W.P., Dobbs, D.B., Keeton, R.E., and Owen, D.G., eds. 1984. Prosser and Keeton on The Law of Torts. St. Paul, Minn.: West.

Mascaro, M.L. 1991. Preconception tort liability: recognizing a strict liability cause of action for DES grandchildren. *American Journal of Law and Medicine* 17(4):435-455.

NIH (National Institutes of Health). 1992. NIH Workshop: Long-Term Effects of Exposure to Diethylstilbestrol (DES), Falls Church, Va., April 22-24, 1992. Sponsored by the Office of Research on Women's Health, National Cancer Institute, National Institute of Child Health and Human Development and the National Institute of Environmental Sciences.

NIH. 1993. RFA CA-93-022, *NIH Guide to Grants and Contracts* 22(15).

Schultz, W. 1982. Inside the courtroom: Illegal experimentation. *Public Citizen* (Spring):28-29.

Squires, S. 1991. DES daughters and their children. *The Washington Post,* February 19:14.

Weitzner, K., and Hirsch, H.L. 1981. Diethylstilbestrol—medicolegal chronology. *Medical Trial Technique Quarterly* 28(Fall):145-170.

## CASE REFERENCES

*Enright v. Eli Lilly & Co.*, 570 N.E.2d 198 (N.Y. 1991).

*Mink v. University of Chicago,* 460 F. Supp. 713 (N.D. Ill. 1978).

*Sorrels v. Eli Lilly & Co.*, 737 F. Supp. 678 (D.D.C. 1990).

*Wetherill v. University of Chicago,* 565 F. Supp. 1553 (N.D. Ill. 1983).

# D

# Compensation Systems
# for Research Injuries

This appendix provides information about compensation systems for research injuries, including: (1) an account of existing compensation systems; (2) the history of past efforts to enact a national system; (3) the issues to be considered when setting up such a system; and (4) lessons to be learned from the experiences of existing compensation systems in the area of medical malpractice.

## EXISTING COMPENSATION SYSTEMS

There is no comprehensive compensation program to cover injuries resulting from privately and publicly funded research. Current federal policy, which applies to federally funded research with "more than minimal risk" to participants, requires that institutions that maintain a compensation system must inform participants of its existence as part of the informed consent process (45 C.F.R. 46.116(a)(6)).

Some institutions have set up their own compensation systems, but many others lack formal policies on compensation but provide acute care for research injuries as a matter of practice. No agency within DHHS, including NIH, currently has a formal compensation policy for injuries resulting from extramural or intramural research. For intramural research, acute care for injuries is routinely provided.

Beyond acute care, however, an injured research participant's only recourse is legal action under the Federal Tort Claims Act (FTCA) (F.W.

Dommel, Office for Protection from Research Risks, personal communication, July 1993). For extramural research, the institutions conducting the research may formulate their own policies regarding compensation, including the option to offer none at all. Most provide acute care for research injuries, but the Office of Protection from Research Risks at NIH knows of no institutions that offer long-term care (F.W. Dommel, Office for Protection from Research Risks, personal communication, July 1993).

Despite the lack of federal guidance in this area, some institutions and pharmaceutical manufacturers have set up compensation systems for research injuries. For example, the University of Washington, the public institution receiving the largest amount of federal biomedical research dollars, has had a liability insurance program that would extend to research injuries in place since 1976.[1] But the University of Washington's program appears to be unique. Most research institutions require participants, as part of the informed consent process, to attest to private insurance coverage of medical costs resulting from research injuries (Kolberg, 1993).

Pharmaceutical manufacturers typically have in-house compensation schemes that pay for medical expenses of injuries directly resulting from drug trials. Pharmaceutical companies also carry liability insurance that would probably reimburse them for loss if a participant brings a successful tort action against them.

## EFFORTS TO DEVELOP A NATIONAL SYSTEM

There has been an ongoing debate since the 1970s about the merits of establishing a compensation system for all participants injured in research (Mariner, 1994). The Public Health Service (PHS) has examined the issue of establishing a compensation system for research injuries over a number of years. In the 1970s, NIH submitted three proposals to the secretary of the Department of Health, Education, and Welfare (HEW)[2] that would have authorized the federal government to indemnify participants in research sponsored in whole or in part by federal funds for any medical and other expenses resulting from research injuries. None of the proposals was accepted.[3] In 1973 an ad hoc panel of the assistant secretary for health (HEW), reviewing the Tuskegee Syphilis Study, recommended a no-fault compensation system (Mariner, 1994). Although no such system was established, HEW reached settlement agreements with all survivors and with some heirs of participants in the Tuskegee study.

In 1975 HEW created a task force to look at compensation for research injuries resulting from federally funded, conducted, and regulated research. The task force recommended that human subjects who suffer physical, psychological, or social injury in the course of research supported by PHS should be compensated if the injury was caused by the research and "the injury on balance exceeds that reasonably associated with such illness from which the subject may be suffering, as well as with treatment usually associated with such illness at the time the subject began participation in research" (HEW, 1977:II-2).

The task force recommended that participants in intramural research be covered by expanding the Federal Employee's Compensation Act (FECA)[4] to include research participants. For extramural research directly supported by PHS, the task force proposed that institutions be required to offer assurance of compensation to each participant, with the compensation to be no less than that provided under FECA. If upon further inquiry the secretary found that it would not be possible for institutions to assure compensation for injured research participants, the task force suggested that FECA be expanded to cover compensation for these participants as well. For research that was regulated but not financially supported by PHS, the task force recommended that the FDA consider legislation that would enable them to require that compensation be made available to injured research participants (HEW, 1977). Drafts of legislation to amend FECA to include participants in research were sent to HEW Secretary Joseph Califano, and proposed regulations to implement the task force's recommendations were also prepared. The same week in August 1979 that Califano was scheduled to sign the proposed rules and forward legislation to the Congress, he was fired by President Carter (Kolberg, 1993). The issue was not picked up by his successor.

After the task force released its report in 1977, the National Commission for the Protection of Human Subjects of Biomedical and Behavioral Research endorsed the recommendations but, without further study, recommended only that subjects be told in the informed consent process whether or not compensation was available (Mariner, 1994).[5]

The secretary of HEW then asked the department's Ethics Advisory Board to look into the recommendations, but the board was dissolved before it could complete the task. Before its termination, the board requested that the President's Commission for the Study of Ethical Problems in Medicine and Biomedical and Behavioral Research continue to consider the issue of compensation. The commission concluded in 1982 that compensation for research injuries was ethically desirable, and suggested that HEW (by now, DHHS) conduct a trial of different forms of compensation systems. Several institutions were to receive federal money over a period of 3-5 years to cover the costs of providing some form of no-fault compensation to injured research subjects (President's Commission for the Study of Ethical Problems in Medicine and Biomedical and Behavioral Research, 1982). Although DHHS considered such experiments, it concluded that they were not feasible and decided not to initiate the trials (C. McCarthy, former director of OPRR, personal communication, July 1993).

Recently there have been more efforts to investigate the possibility of compensation for injured research participants. In January 1993, the Recombinant DNA Advisory Committee (RAC) sent a letter to NIH Director Bernadine Healy, asking her to form a panel to look at covering medical costs of research-related, nonnegligent injuries. The letter stated that it was "unfair to expect individuals, their families, or their insurers to absorb unpredictable and potentially substantial medical costs arising out of these individuals' participation as research subjects" (Walters, 1993a). In a subsequent letter, the RAC appealed to Dr. Healy to ask the health care reform task force to address the issue of providing health care coverage for persons who are injured as a result of participating in clinical research (Walters, 1993b).

The effort to investigate compensation for research injuries is not limited to the United States. Although countries with national health care systems generally do not face the same pressures to create a separate compensation system for research injuries (President's Commission, 1982), nevertheless two major international health organizations developed compensation recommendations. The same year the commission released its report, the World Health Organization (WHO) and the Council for International Organizations of Medical Sciences (CIOMS) issued their guidelines for human subjects research, which declared that volunteer subjects are entitled to full compensation for temporary or permanent disability or death.

These guidelines also recommended that pharmaceutical manufacturers assume responsibility for injuries resulting from research they sponsor. A recently revised version of these guidelines (1993) states that every subject is entitled to equitable compensation, except for expected adverse reactions from investigational interventions to diagnose or prevent disease (Mariner, 1994).

## ISSUES IN DEVELOPING
## A NATIONAL COMPENSATION SYSTEM

Professor Mariner, in her paper published in Volume 2 of this report, discusses a variety of compensation systems for research injuries and their advantages and disadvantages. Advantages of a federal compensation program include the ability of injured parties to get benefits more easily, because they are not required to go into court and prove fault; usually, they need only show plausible evidence that their injuries were research-related. Other advantages include a higher percentage of injured participants and offspring receiving compensation, as well as a higher percentage of each compensation award going directly to the injured party.

In addition, the costs to administer the system are far less than those of litigation. These costs may be spread over all who benefit from the research enterprise, particularly if the program is funded through general tax revenues (Mariner, 1994).

Disadvantages to a compensation system include the difficulty that some claimants may have showing the causal relationship between their injuries and the research. This would be particularly relevant in the case of offspring injuries, where causation is often nearly impossible to prove. In addition, the existence of a compensation system may result in more people making claims under the system than would have otherwise pursued recovery through the courts. This may indicate a real need for the program; but it may also result in an unjustifiable rise in program costs, because people can misjudge the cause of their injuries (Mariner, 1994).

The issues to be considered in developing a compensation system are numerous and complex. One crucial issue that must be resolved is determining *who* and *what* gets compensated (Mariner, 1994). For example, should the compensation system be available to all research participants, or only those participating in research for which they receive no health benefits? The issues are arguably more complex if offspring injured by a parent's participation in a clinical trial are to be included in the system. For example, if the parent consented to research after being adequately informed, is an offspring injury still eligible for compensation? Would the system cover injuries to offspring in protocols where the parent agreed to use contraception, and subsequently used inadequate contraception or none at all?

Once it is determined *who* is to be compensated, the next question is: *what* injuries will be eligible for compensation? The resolution of this issue is particularly important for offspring injuries, because their injuries are often discovered many years after the research protocol is complete. The section below discusses three specific examples of compensation systems set up to alleviate medical malpractice concerns, and it demonstrates the relative advantages and disadvantages between setting up a system with a broad base of compensable events and restricting the system to specific types of injuries.

Another important feature of any compensation system is the extent of the benefits available to eligible participants. The current tort system provides the most generous compensation available, with benefits ranging from recompense for physical injuries and lost wages to pain and suffering and, occasionally, punitive damages (Abraham, 1988). But since a compensation system offers some benefit to the participant in the rapid recovery of damages with administratively easy procedures, the participant is in turn asked to forego full recovery. The resolution of the question of benefits requires a compromise between the desire to be fair to the participant and the need to create a system that will remain fiscally solvent over time. Any compensation system necessarily limits recovery relative to what a plaintiff could gain pursuing a claim through the tort system, which creates some question of horizontal justice: persons suffering injury from other causes can recover full tort damages, whereas those injured through research are entitled to limited recovery (Abraham, 1988). This concern would be alleviated, however, by allowing injured research participants to elect the system in which to pursue recovery. In addition, a decision must be made about whether the system will be applied retroactively or only to prospective participants (Mariner, 1994).

A related issue to the scope of benefits is the payment mechanism. Built into any compensation system is a structure for paying out benefits. Under a third-party insurance scheme, groups and individuals involved in the conduct of research would be required to obtain private insurance to cover research injuries. If a system requires first-party insurance, the participant is required to purchase insurance before entering a clinical study. Under a social insurance system, the government would insure or reinsure individuals or groups conducting research against the costs of research injuries. Finally, patient compensation funds could serve as the available pool of money for compensating research injuries, for which contributions may be exacted from the various groups involved in the conduct of research (Abraham, 1988).

How the system would be administered is also a critical consideration. To some extent it will be governed by the payment mechanism selected. For example, a third- or first-party insurance-based system will likely be administered by an insurance company. If the system is government-sponsored, an agency will need to be set up to handle the claims. Within issues of administration are concerns about the participants' right to appeal any decisions not to compensate (Mariner, 1994).

Although in theory the creation of a compensation system for research injuries appears to be a worthwhile endeavor, it is by no means an uncomplicated solution. As demonstrated above, the complexities involved in setting up a compensation system are numerous, and decisions made in structuring the system have direct implications for how fairly the compensation system will meet the burden of research injuries.

## EXAMPLES OF COMPENSATION SYSTEMS IN THE AREA OF MEDICAL MALPRACTICE

The debate about tort reform in the area of medical malpractice has been an active one for more than a decade. Given the similarity in legal issues between medical malpractice and liability for research injuries, examples of medical malpractice reform efforts may be particularly instructive to any consideration of a compensation system for research injuries. This section discusses the advantages and disadvantages of three examples:

the birth injury compensation systems in Virginia and Florida, and the National Vaccine Injury Compensation Act.

## Virginia and Florida

During the late 1980s, legislatures in Virginia and Florida enacted narrowly circumscribed no-fault compensation schemes to alleviate insurer concern about particularly high damage awards in cases where infants sustained severe, disabling neurological injury during the delivery process.

Under the Virginia Birth-Related Neurological Injury Compensation Act (Va. Code §§ 38.2-5000 et seq. [1990 Real. Vol.]), an infant sustaining "birth-related neurological injury," as defined in the act, is entitled to payment for medical, rehabilitative, and residential expenses not recoverable from any governmental program or private insurance. The infant also receives reasonable expenses of filing a claim and a scheduled amount for loss of earnings between ages 18 and 65. Eligibility for compensation also depends on whether a child was delivered by a "participating physician" or in a "participating hospital." Damages are not recoverable for pain and suffering. In circumstances where the act applies, the remedies it provides are exclusive, supplanting the tort system.

One distinguishing element to Virginia's system is its very limited applicability. Even after an amendment that broadened the act's original definition of "birth-related neurological injury," it remains very limited in scope. In addition, the act requires that the disability must cause the infant to be "permanently in need of assistance in all activities of daily living." As a result of the narrow scope of coverage, by mid-1993 only four claims had been paid under the Virginia Act.

The Virginia scheme is financed through annually assessing physicians and hospitals, with possible surcharges against insurers should that become necessary. Currently *every* physician in the state is assessed $250 annually.[6] "Participating physicians" pay $5,000 and "participating hospitals" pay according to the number of live births in their facility during the previous year.

Florida's no-fault compensation scheme was modeled largely on the Virginia law. Its definition of "injury" is different, however, and far more claims have been paid under Florida's act, even though it has been in operation for less time. This may well be not only because of the somewhat less restrictive definition but also because Florida provides for a lump-sum payment of as much as $100,000. All hospitals are required participants under the Florida act.

## National Childhood Vaccine Injury Act

The National Childhood Vaccine Injury Act (42 U.S.C.A. § 300aa-1 to -33 [1989]) was enacted by Congress to provide payments to children suffering harm through vaccine-related accidents on a "no-fault" basis. The ostensible purpose was to assure that vaccine production would continue. Before passage of the act, the costs of liability for vaccine-related injuries were grossly out of proportion to the profits manufacturers derived from the sale of vaccines. Under the act, an injured party must first file a claim with the Department of Health and Human Services. The injuries eligible for compensation are strictly prescribed, and the likelihood of receiving compensation depends on whether the injury appears in the Vaccine Injury Table.

The major advantage of the act is that once a claimant demonstrates an injury from the Vaccine Injury Table, he or she is eligible to receive compensation for damages; there is no need to show that anyone was negligent. The damages are limited, however, including only actual costs of treatment not covered by public or private insurance and attorneys' fees, with caps on damages for pain and suffering (Clayton and Hickson, 1990). Children whose injuries do not appear in the table must show that the vaccine actually caused their injuries, which can be difficult to prove. If a compensation award is offered and the family accepts it, they may not pursue a legal action in tort against the vaccine manufacturer or the physician. If the family chooses not to accept the award (or if the claim is rejected as ineligible for compensation), the family may pursue recovery through the tort system (Clayton and Hickson, 1990).

The advantages of the act include the guarantee of some measure of recovery for eligible children, without the delays and often prohibitive requirements of the tort system—for example, the need to prove negligence. Because of the choice to limit the compensable injuries, however, there may be injured children who receive no compensation. In addition, the Congressional Budget Office estimates that 220 vaccine-related injuries occur each year (Clayton and Hickson, 1990, citing H. Rep. No. 100-391, 100th Cong., 1st Sess. 693-4 [1987]). But there is a limit of 150 awards a year, which means that the act will lapse unless Congress steps in to provide more funds (Clayton and Hickson, 1990). Thus, there is reason to be concerned that the system could collapse under the weight of eligible claims.

### NOTES

1. The coverage, provided on a no-fault basis, has an upper limit of $10,000, is limited to expenses from physical injuries, and applies only to injuries to healthy, normal participants (H. McGough, Human Subjects Di-

vision, University of Washington, personal communication, June 1993). As a condition of accepting reimbursement for physical injuries, the participant waives the right to seek legal action in tort against the university. In the past five years there have only been three or four claims for compensation, and the university has paid less than $2,000 in compensation for injuries (E. Cherry, Risk Management Office, University of Washington, personal communication, June 1993).

2.   The health and welfare components of HEW are now the Department of Health and Human Services (DHHS).

3.   The proposals were rejected for one or more of the following reasons: the social and fiscal implications of the proposal had not been adequately investigated, alternatives to a federal compensation program had not been examined, and the extent of the problem had not been fully defined (HEW, 1977).

4.   FECA is the statute that specifies limited levels of compensation for federal employees who are injured in the course of their work.

5.   This recommendation was incorporated into the federal regulations governing human subjects research (45 C.F.R. section 46.116(a)(6)).

6.   There are exceptions for retired physicians and others working in free clinics. See Va. Code section 38.2-5020.D (Cum. Sup. 1992).

## REFERENCES

Abraham, K.S. 1988. Medical liability reform: A conceptual framework. *Journal of the American Medical Association* 260(1):68-72.

Cherry, E. 1993. Conversation of D. McGraw with E. Cherry, head of risk management office, University of Washington. June 1993.

Clayton, E.W., Hickson, G.B. 1990. Compensation under the National Childhood Vaccine Injury Act. *The Journal of Pediatrics* 116(4):508-513.

Dommel, W. 1993. Conversation of D. McGraw with William Dommel of NIH on compensation for research injuries (July 6).

Edwards, L.D. 1992. Design and Conduct of Research in Women: To Include or Exclude: A Pharmaceutical Industry Physician's Perspective. Monograph prepared for NIH Office of Protection from Research Risks.

HEW Secretary's Task Force on the Compensation of Injured Research Subjects. 1977. Washington, D.C. U.S. Department of Health, Education and Welfare (HEW).

Kolberg, R. 1993. RAC asks, who should pay for research injuries? *The Journal of NIH Research* 5(February):36-38.

Mariner, W.K. 1994. Compensation for research injuries. In: Women and Health Research: Ethical and Legal Issues of Including Women in Clinical Studies, Volume 2, A. Mastroianni, R. Faden, and D. Federman, eds., Washington, D.C.: National Academy Press.

McCarthy, C. 1993. Personal communication by D. McGraw with C. McCarthy, former director, Office of Protection from Research Risks (July).

McGough, H. 1993. Conversation of D. McGraw with H. McGough, Human Subjects Division, University of Washington (June).

President's Commission for the Study of Ethical Problems in Medicine and Biomedical and Behavioral Research. 1982. Compensating for Research Injuries: A Report on the Ethical and Legal Implications of Programs to Redress Injuries Caused by Biomedical and Behavioral Research. Volume 1. Washington, D.C.: Government Printing Office.

Walters, L.B. 1993a. Letter from Dr. LeRoy B. Walters, Chair, Recombinant DNA Advisory Committee, to Dr. Bernadine Healy, Director, National Institutes of Health. January 6, 1993.

Walters, L.B. 1993b. Letter from Dr. LeRoy B. Walters, Chair, Recombinant DNA Advisory Committee, to Dr. Bernadine Healy, Director, National Institutes of Health. June 28, 1993.

## STATUTORY AND REGULATORY REFERENCES

42 USCA §300aa-1 to -33 (1989)
45 C.F.R. 46.116(a)(b)
Va. Code Sections 38.2-5000 et seq. [1990 Real. Vol.]

# E

# Committee Biographies

**Ruth Faden,** Ph.D., M.P.H., is Professor and Director of the Program in Law, Ethics, and Health at the Johns Hopkins University School of Hygiene and Public Health. She is also Senior Research Scholar at the Kennedy Institute of Ethics at Georgetown University. Dr. Faden received her Ph.D. in 1976 and her M.P.H. in 1973, both from the University of California at Berkeley. She is a member of the American Association of Bioethics and the American Psychological Association, and has served on the Governing Council of the American Public Health Association. Dr. Faden has also served on a number of advisory committees, including those for the National Academy of Sciences, Social Science Research Council, Office of Technology Assessment, National Institutes of Health, Centers for Disease Control, and as a consultant to the National Commission for the Protection of Human Subjects of Biomedical and Behavioral Research and the President's Commission for the Study of Ethical Problems in Medicine and Biomedical and Behavioral Research. She has authored numerous articles and books, including *AIDS, Women and the Next Generation* and *A History and Theory of Informed Consent* (Oxford University Press, 1986 and 1991)

**Daniel Federman,** M.D., was graduated from Harvard College and Harvard Medical School and had his internship and residency at Massachusetts General Hospital. He conducted research and trained in endocrinology at the National Institutes of Health, the University College Hospital Medical School in London, and Massachusetts General Hospital. He has served as Physician, Chief of the Endocrine Unit, and Associate Chief of Medical Services at the Massachusetts General Hospital and was later Arthur F. Bloomfield Professor of Medicine and Chairman of the Department of Medicine at Stanford University Medical School. Since 1977 Dr. Federman has served as Dean for Students and Alumni and Professor of Medicine at Harvard Medical School. He is currently Dean for Medical Education and the Carl W. Walter Professor of Medicine and Medical Education. Dr. Federman has served as Chairman of the Board of Internal Medicine and President of the American College of Physicians. He is a member of the Institute of Medicine.

**Anita Allen,** J.D., Ph.D., is Professor of Law at the Georgetown University Law Center. She received her J.D. from Harvard Law School in 1984 and her Ph.D. in philosophy from the University of Michigan in 1979. She has also served as Visiting Professor of Law at Harvard Law School and Distinguished Visiting Adjunct Professor of Philosophy and Women's Studies at the University of Pennsylvania. Professor Allen is a member of several professional organizations, including the American Association of Law School Teachers, the American Association of University Professors, the American Bar Association, and the American Society for Political and Legal Philosophy. She has published several book chapters and articles and has spoken at numerous conferences and seminars. Professor Allen is admitted to the bar in New York and Pennsylvania.

**Hortensia Amaro,** Ph.D., is Professor of Social and Behavioral Sciences in the School of Public Health at Boston University. She received her doctorate in developmental and social psychology in 1982 from the University of California at Los Angeles. She has served as a consultant and in various advisory roles to the Surgeon General's Agenda on Hispanic Health, the Centers for Disease Control, the National Institutes of Health, the National Institute on Drug Abuse, and the Center for Substance Abuse Prevention, as well as to foundations and community-based organizations. She is founder and past president of the Latino Health Institute of Massachusetts and founder of the Multicultural AIDS Coalition and the National Hispanic Psychological Association. She has received numerous awards including the Alfred Frechette Award from the Massachusetts Public Health Association, and the American Psychological Association's Early Career Award for Contributions to Psychology in the Public Interest. She serves as associate editor for the *Psychology of Women Quarterly* and on the editorial board of the *American Journal of Public Health*. Dr. Amaro's research has focused on epidemiological studies and community-based interventions for substance abuse and HIV among women, and on Hispanic health issues.

**Karen H. Antman,** M.D., is Professor of Medicine and Chief, Division of Medical Oncology, Columbia University. Dr. Antman received her M.D. from Columbia University's College of Physicians and Surgeons. She joined the Harvard Medical School faculty in 1979 and served as the Clinical Director of the Dana-Farber Cancer Institute and Beth Israel Hospital Solid Tumor Autologous Marrow Program and coordinated the sarcoma and mesothelioma clinical research and treatment programs at the Dana-Farber Cancer Institute until 1993. She is an Associate Editor of the *New England Journal of Medicine* and is on the editorial board of *Annals of Internal Medicine.* She has consulted for the U.S. Department of Justice on asbestos-related malignancies and has served on the Health and Human Services Advisory Board, Study of Coverage for Investigational Therapy and the Physicians Payment Review Commission/American Medical Association Consensus Panel for Evaluation and Management of Services (both in 1989), and on the Harvard Resources Based Relative Value Scale Technical Consulting Panel from 1989 to 1990. She has served on the Board of Directors of the American Society of Clinical Oncology (ASCO) and was Chairman of the Public Issues Committee for the past four years, repeatedly testifying before congressional committees. She is currently President-elect of ASCO. She is an author on more than 100 original reports, 5 editorials, 67 review articles or textbook chapters, and has edited or written 3 textbooks and monographs.

**Lionel D. Edwards,** MBBS, FFPM, DObst, RCOG, graduated from Guy's Hospital Medical School, London University, and worked in Family Practice, with part-time appointments in Rheumatology and Obstetrics. After 7 years of clinical practice, he joined the pharmaceutical industry, where over the last 19 years he has held various international and U.S. director positions in Clinical Research operations at Roussel, Upjohn, Abbott, Schering Plough Research Institute, and Hoffmann-La Roche. He has been heavily involved in contributing key studies to the Food and Drug Administration and international regulatory authorities on allergy, antibiotic, oncology, cardiovascular, and OTC products. He is Assistant Vice President, International Clinical Research, Hoffmann-La Roche. He is Chairman of the Pharmaceutical Manufacturers Association (PMA) Special Populations Committee and teaches in three different courses for PMA/PERI, and is the PMA ICH representative for the Orlando ICH II meeting for workshop topic 5—Ethnic Factors in the Acceptability of Foreign Data.

**Ann Barry Flood,** Ph.D., is Director of Policy Studies and Associate Professor at the Center for the Evaluative Clinical Sciences at Dartmouth Medical School. She received her doctorate in Organizational Sociology from Stanford University in 1977. She also served on the staff of the U.S.

Senate Finance Committee during 1989 as a Robert Wood Johnson Health Policy Fellow. Dr. Flood's areas of theoretical and policy expertise involve understanding the professional and organizational factors that influence physicians' styles of practice, patients' outcomes, and the costs of health care.

**Shiriki K. Kumanyika,** Ph.D., M.P.H., is Professor of Epidemiology and Associate Director for Epidemiology at the Pennsylvania State University College of Medicine (Milton S. Hershey Medical Center). She earned her M.S. (1969) in Social Work from Columbia University, a Ph.D. (1978) in Human Nutrition from Cornell University, and an M.P.H. (1984) in Epidemiology from Johns Hopkins University. Before coming to Penn State in 1989 with a primary appointment in nutrition (1989-1992), Dr. Kumanyika held faculty positions in Nutrition and Epidemiology, respectively, at Cornell University and Johns Hopkins University. She is currently principal investigator of a National Institutes of Health (NIH) grant to develop cardiovascular education materials for black American adults with low literacy skills and is a co-investigator on two multicenter trials for hypertension prevention or treatment. Her publications reflect 16 years of research related to cardiovascular diseases, obesity, nutritional epidemiology, and the health of minority populations, older populations, and women. Dr. Kumanyika currently chairs the National Nutrition Monitoring Advisory Council and serves or has served on several other national task forces and advisory committees, including the NIH Behavioral Medicine Study Section, the NIH Epidemiology and Disease Control Study Section, the NIH Office of Women's Health Research Task Forces on Opportunities for Research in Women's Health and on the Recruitment and Retention of Women in Clinical Studies (which she co-chairs), and the Women's Health Initiative Policy Advisory Committee.

**Ruth Macklin,** Ph.D. is a Professor in the Department of Epidemiology and Social Medicine at Albert Einstein College of Medicine. She received a B.A. with distinction from Cornell University, and her M.A. and Ph.D. in philosophy from Case Western Reserve University. She has had more than 120 publications in professional journals and scholarly books in philosophy, bioethics, and law and medicine, in addition to articles in magazines and newspapers for general audiences. She is author or editor of seven books, including *Mortal Choices*, published by Houghton Mifflin in 1988 and *Enemies of Patients*, published by Oxford University Press in 1993. Her writings explore ethical issues in the clinical practice of medicine, biomedical and behavioral research involving human subjects, health policy, and health law. She is a member of the Institute of Medicine of the National Academy of Sciences, and is a consultant to and board member of several national and international organizations, including the National Institutes of Health, the National Research Council, and the World Health Organization.

**Donald R. Mattison,** M.D. is Dean of the Graduate School of Public Health and Professor of Environmental and Occupational Health and Obstetrics and Gynecology at the University of Pittsburgh. Dr. Mattison received his undergraduate education at Augsburg College, where he majored in Chemistry and Mathematics, and an M.S. in Chemistry from the Massachusetts Institute of Technology. He received his M.D. from The College of Physicians and Surgeons, Columbia University, and clinical training in obstetrics and gynecology at Sloane Hospital for Women, Columbia Presbyterian Medical Center, in New York. Dr. Mattison obtained postgraduate research training at the National Institutes of Health. From 1978 to 1984 Dr. Mattison was director of the Reproductive Toxicology Program in the Pregnancy Research Branch, National Institute of Child Health and Human Development, National Institutes of Health. From 1984 to 1990 he was Professor of Obstetrics and Gynecology and Toxicology at the University of Arkansas for Medical Sciences. During this period he was also Acting Director of the Human Risk Assessment Program at the National Center for Toxicological Research, a component of the Food and Drug Administration. Dr. Mattison has been at the University of Pittsburgh since August of 1990. Dr. Mattison is a member of many local and national boards. He has published more than 140 papers, chapters, and reviews in the areas of reproductive and developmental toxicology, risk assessment, and clinical obstetrics and gynecology.

**Charles R. McCarthy,** Ph.D., is Senior Research Fellow, Kennedy Institute of Ethics, Georgetown University. Trained in philosophy and political science at the University of Toronto, Dr. McCarthy taught at The Catholic University of America and George Washington University. Employed by the National Institutes of Health (NIH) in 1971, he functioned as Chief of the Legislative Development Branch and Executive Secretary of the NIH Director's Advisory Committee. In 1978 he was appointed Staff Director of the Secretary's Ethics Advisory Board. For the final 14 years of his career at the NIH he served as Director of the Office for Protection from Research Risks. In this capacity he was responsible for providing protection for human research subjects throughout the United States and in 80 nations worldwide, and for the humane care and use of laboratory animals. Dr. McCarthy has written many articles and received a number of honors including the Outstanding Achievement Award from the Secretary of Health and Human Services. Currently he is a member of the Board of Directors of Public Responsibility in Medicine and Research, of the Board of Directors of the Scientists Center for Animal Welfare, of the Ethics Committee of the American Fertility Society, and serves as Ethics Staff Consultant to the Acadia Institute.

**Curtis L. Meinert,** Ph.D., is Director of the Center for Clinical Trials at the Johns Hopkins University School of Hygiene and Public Health, where he is also a Professor of Epidemiology and Biostatistics. He received his Ph.D. in Biostatistics from the University of Minnesota in 1964. Throughout his career he has been involved in the design and conduct of more than 20 clinical trials, starting with the University Group Diabetes Program in the 1960s. Recently, he has served as Director of the Coordinating Centers for the Glaucoma Laser Trial and the Hypertension Prevention Trial. He currently heads the Coordinating Center for Studies of Ocular Complications of AIDS. He was a founding member of the Society for Clinical Trials, served on its first Board of Directors, and has been editor of its journal, *Controlled Clinical Trials*, since its inception in 1980. Dr. Meinert is the Director of the Clinical Trial Training Program and is the co-author of a textbook, *Clinical Trials: Design, Conduct, and Analysis* (1986, Oxford University Press). His teaching activities include a basic course on the design, conduct, and analysis of clinical trials and numerous intensive, short courses given both on the Johns Hopkins campuses and off campus at governmental agencies located in the Washington, D.C., area. He has been active on the Institutional Review Boards for both the Johns Hopkins Medical School and the School of Hygiene and Public Health and is currently Chair of the Committee on Human Research for the latter. In addition, he has served on advisory review committees and treatment effects monitoring committees for numerous trials both in this country and internationally. Dr. Meinert has also served on numerous National Academy of Science committees. He was also a member of the National Institutes of Health Task Force on Population-Based Research Training. Dr. Meinert has served as a consultant to governmental agencies and private industry and recently was an expert witness for the Federal Trade Commission.

**Karen H. Rothenberg,** J.D., M.P.A., is Professor of Law, the M. Jacqueline McCurdy Scholar, and Director of the Law and Health Care Program at the University of Maryland School of Law. She received her B.A., *magna cum laude,* and her M.P.A. from Princeton University, and a J.D. from the University of Virginia. She formerly practiced with the D.C. Law firm of Covington and Burling and has worked a variety of health and medical organizations including serving as legal counsel to the American College of Nurse-Midwives and on a number of National Institutes of Health panels. She is 1993-1994 president of the American Society of Law, Medicine and Ethics. Professor Rothenberg has written numerous articles on AIDS, women's health, genetic testing, the right to forego treatment, emergency care, and surrogacy, and lectures extensively on legal issues in health care.

**Anthony R. Scialli,** M.D., is Director of the Residency Program in Obstetrics and Gynecology at Georgetown University Medical Center and is

Director of the Reproductive Toxicology Center at Columbia Hospital for Women Medical Center, Washington, D.C. He received his M.D. at Albany Medical College and completed a residency in obstetrics and gynecology at George Washington University, following which he took a fellowship in reproductive toxicology with the late Sergio Fabro. Dr. Scialli is the founder and editor-in-chief of the journal *Reproductive Toxicology* and author of *A Clinical Guide to Reproductive and Developmental Toxicology*. He has served as a consultant to several government and private organizations on the effects of chemical and physical agents on reproduction, and is an active teacher and researcher in the field of teratology and reproductive toxicology.

**Sheldon J. Segal,** Ph.D., is a Distinguished Scientist at the Population Council in New York City and was Director for Population Sciences at the Rockefeller Foundation from 1978 through 1991. A Dartmouth graduate, he received his Ph.D. in Embryology and Biochemistry from the University of Iowa and is the recipient of honorary M.D. degrees from the University of Uppsala, Sweden, and the University of Tampere, Finland. Dr. Segal is a senior member of the Institute of Medicine and an honorary member of the Mexican Academy of Medicine and of the Chinese Academy of Sciences. The 1984 Laureate of the United Nations Population Award, he is a leading authority on global population issues, family planning, and contraceptive technology. Dr. Segal serves as advisor to the World Health Organization's Safe Motherhood Programme and is an Adjunct Professor, Department of Pharmacology, Cornell University Medical College. He is Chairman of the Board of Trustees, Marine Biological Laboratory, Woods Hole, Massachusetts, and a Director of the Center for Reproductive Law and Policy.

**Walter J. Wadlington,** LL.B. is James Madison Professor of Law at the University of Virginia School of Law and Professor of Legal Medicine at the University of Virginia School of Medicine. He was the Program Director of the Robert Wood Johnson Foundation Medical Malpractice Program. He is a member of the Institute of Medicine, the American Law Institute, and the Advisory Committee of the Robert Wood Johnson Clinical Scholars Program. Mr. Wadlington teaches in the areas of law and medicine, family law, and children's health care.

# Index

## A

Abortion, 12, 119, 144
  discussed during consent procedure, 15, 193, 194
Abuses by researchers, *see* Unethical treatment
Access to research
  policy development, 2, 36, 37, 42-43, 69
  registry information, 3, 4, 69, 70
Accountability for policy implementation, 19, 203, 205
Acquired immune deficiency syndrome, *see* AIDS
Adenosis, 238
Adipose tissue, 86
Adverse reactions, 16, 89, 131, 140, 189
  and compensation, 152, 246
  liability issues, 12, 150, 165-167
  *see also* Prenatal and preconceptual injury
Advocacy and activism, 1, 2, 37, 42-43, 69, 121, 192

African Americans, 117
  research abuses of, 38, 39, 76, 118, 121
  *see also* Tuskegee Syphilis Study
Age and age groups, 5, 23, 77, 82, 83, 99, 119-120, 209
  database information on, 4, 24, 70
  *see also* Aging and the elderly; Menopause and postmenopausal women; Reproductive and childbearing potential
Aging and the elderly, 89-90, 120, 185
  research abuses and inequity, 38, 44, 54, 66, 220
  *see also* Menopause and postmenopausal women
AIDS, 37, 54, 56, 59, 143, 220-221, 223-224, 228-229
  activism and advocacy, 2, 31, 37, 42-43
  inequity in studies of, 3, 49, 55, 56, 66, 78, 80-81, 112, 222, 223
Alaskan natives, 116, 117, 118
Alcohol, Drug Abuse, and Mental Health Administration, 43, 70$n$

# M

Magnesium sulfate, 188
Male bias, 8, 110, 111-112
Male norm, 8-9, 80, 110, 113-114
Mania, 90
Maternity, *see* Pregnancy; Prenatal and preconceptual injury
Men
  DES injuries of, 238
  and justice in research, 5, 23, 77, 78, 80, 82
  registry inclusion of, 3, 69
  reproductive risks to, 12, 14-15, 138, 162, 175, 178, 179, 181, 182, 193
  *see also* Male bias; Male norm; *terms beginning with* Gender
Menopause and postmenopausal women, 5-6, 94-95
  disease prevention study, 45
  heart disease, 64, 65-66, 78
Menstrual cycle, 5, 91, 111, 113, 120, 140-141
  DES-related irregularity, 238
Mental health problems, 90
Meta-analysis, 101-102, 135
Metabolism, 86
Methodological issues, 8, 9, 10, 24-25, 95-103, 114-117, 125
  in policy compliance, 24, 211
Methyl mercury, 179
Minimal risk, 142, 163
Minority groups, *see* Race and ethnicity
Miscarriage, 179
  and DES, 237
Model Federal Policy, 141-142
Monetary inducement, 10, 82, 122, 125
Monitoring, of policy compliance, 19, 21, 22, 206
  *see also* Surveillance and monitoring
Multicenter studies, 4, 69
Multiple Risk-Factor Intervention Trials (MRFIT), 44, 51, 65, 99, 100, 217

# N

National Childhood Vaccine Injury Act, 250
National Commission for the Protection of Human Subjects of Biomedical and Behavioral Research, 4, 41, 75, 245
National Institutes of Health (NIH), 10, 11, 27, 129-130
  failure to implement inclusion policy, 2, 43, 47-48
  investigator training and education, 9, 10, 11-12, 21, 45, 125, 207
  lack of injury compensation policies, 243
  legal actions against, 151, 157-158, 170*n*
  policy consistency and congruence, 11, 167-168
  policy implementation and guidance, 22, 23-25, 45, 105, 132-137, 193, 203-211 *passim*
  recommended studies, 7, 8, 10, 23, 105, 210, 211
  registry implementation and use, 2, 47, 67-68, 70
  *see also* Office of Protection from Research Risks; Office of Research on Women's Health
National Institutes of Health (NIH) Revitalization Act, 2, 27, 44-45, 135-137, 233-236
  registry provision, 3, 47, 68, 69, 136
  representative sample provision, 2-3, 7, 9-10, 24-25, 104, 114, 119, 125, 132-133, 135-137, 147, 204
National Library of Medicine (NLM), 68, 129
National Research Act, 41
National research agenda, 1, 2, 4, 37, 69
  principles of justice in, 5, 22-23, 77, 78, 81, 82, 204, 209
Nazis, 37, 68, 76
Negligence, 153-154, 156, 168-169
Neurodegenerative diseases, 90